Aesthetic Clinic Marketing in the Digital Age

Aesthetic practitioners and medical spas have flourished, and global statistics indicate that consumer engagement is at an all-time high. The rise of social media provides new ways to connect with consumers and differentiate clinics that stand out in the marketplace. For busy clinic managers and practitioners, keeping up with the nuances of digital media trends is practically a full-time job. With over 25 years of experience in medical aesthetics, Wendy Lewis shares her deep understanding of the challenges aesthetic practitioners face to effectively market their products and services, manage patients, and increase profits. This updated text is the definitive expert user's guide written specifically for healthcare professionals and medical spa managers to present best practices and actionable strategies for mastering digital marketing, social media, branding, and the advent of AI. It is a must-read for aesthetic practitioners to keep up with the latest developments they need to manage their businesses effectively in this highly competitive field.

This second edition features:

- NEW chapters on hot topics you need to know
- MORE tips, charts, tables, and resources
- UP-TO-THE-MINUTE strategies for success

T0313235

Aesthetic Clinic Marketing in the Digital Age

From Meta to AI

Second Edition

Wendy Lewis

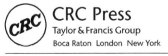

CRC Press
Taylor & Francis Group
Boca Raton London New York

CRC Press is an imprint of the
Taylor & Francis Group, an **informa** business

Designed cover image: Shutterstock

Second edition published 2024
by CRC Press
2385 NW Executive Center Drive, Suite 320, Boca Raton, FL 33431

and by CRC Press
4 Park Square, Milton Park, Abingdon, Oxon, OX14 4RN

CRC Press is an imprint of Taylor & Francis Group, LLC

© 2024 Taylor & Francis Group, LLC

Library of Congress Cataloging-in-Publication Data
Names: Lewis, Wendy, 1959- author.
Title: Aesthetic clinic marketing in the digital age : from Meta to AI /
Wendy Lewis.
Description: Second. | Boca Raton : CRC Press, 2024. | Includes
bibliographical references and index. | Summary: "It's a brave new
world. Aesthetic practitioners and medical spas have flourished, and
global statistics indicate that consumer engagement is at an all-time
high. The rise of social media provides new ways to connect with
consumers to differentiate their clinics and stand out in the
marketplace. For busy clinic managers and practitioners, keeping up with
the nuances of digital media trends is practically a full-time job. With
over 25 years of experience in medical aesthetics, Lewis shares her deep
understanding of the challenges they face to effectively market their
products and services, manage patients, and increase profits. This
updated text is the definitive expert user's guide written specifically
for healthcare professionals and medical spa managers to present best
practices and actionable strategies for mastering digital marketing,
social media, branding, and the advent of AI. It is a must-read for
aesthetic practitioners to keep up with the latest developments they
need to manage their businesses effectively in this highly competitive
field. This second edition features: New chapters on hot topics you need
to know, More tips, charts, tables, and resources, and Up to the minute
strategies for success"-- Provided by publisher.
Identifiers: LCCN 2024000061 (print) | LCCN 2024000062 (ebook) | ISBN
9780367405656 (hardback) | ISBN 9780367405182 (paperback) | ISBN
9780429356742 (ebook)
Subjects: MESH: Cosmetic Techniques--economics | Beauty Culture--economics
| Marketing of Health Services | Social Media--economics
Classification: LCC TT965 (print) | LCC TT965 (ebook) | NLM WO 595 | DDC
646.7/2068--dc23/eng/20240202
LC record available at https://lccn.loc.gov/2024000061
LC ebook record available at https://lccn.loc.gov/2024000062

ISBN: 9780367405656 (hbk)
ISBN: 9780367405182 (pbk)
ISBN: 9780429356742 (ebk)

DOI: 10.1201/9780429356742

Typeset in Times
by Deanta Global Publishing Services, Chennai, India

Dedication

I have dedicated all ten books I have penned in my own name throughout my career

to my amazing daughter, Eden Claire Lipke-Weiss. I am a very proud mom!

She is the light of my life and the smartest, most talented, switched-on social strategist

and strategic marketer I know. I take no credit for her success; she did it 100% on

her own. I am delighted that she has found her soulmate Jordan Weiss.

I also want to thank and acknowledge my editor, Robert Peden at Taylor & Francis, who has been

more patient and forgiving with me than any author ever deserved to get this book into print!

And finally, a huge thank you to the colleagues who have supported me through this

journey: Heidi Martiak, Rachel DelPozo, Denise Kleinman, Sheila Shiels, Ran Berkman,

Anne Lindley, plus a shout out for my #1 writing partner, Remy the Havanese.

Contents

Preface

This is my tenth book to be published since I founded my company, Wendy Lewis & Co Ltd, Global Aesthetics Consultancy, in 1997. The first eight books I penned in my own name were written for consumers interested in learning about the latest and greatest trends in beauty treatments, cosmetic surgery, and making good choices. I have also helped many physicians craft their own books and have contributed to a handful of medical textbooks as well. The first book I wrote, *Facelifts and Other Wrinkle Remedies*, was published by Quadrille Publishing in 2001 and serialized in the *Daily Mail*. My ninth book and the first textbook I wrote for professionals is titled *Aesthetic Clinic Marketing in the Digital Age*, from CRC Press, and is still in circulation. I have also served as a ghostwriter for multiple books for physicians, one of which made *The New York Times* Best Seller List, and all of which shall remain nameless.

I started writing this new edition before the pandemic turned our whole world upside down. In retrospect, I am glad that I waited to finalize this manuscript at this time, after witnessing so many shifts in medical aesthetics globally. I have been encouraged by many practitioners, nurses, practice managers, and booksellers who I have met at congresses all over the world asking when my next book was coming.

The greatest challenge for me in finalizing this book was squeezing it into my busy workload for our clients and frequent travel commitments, as well as the monthly array of articles I write for multiple publications. I have been honored to have been invited by six leading physicians, plastic surgeons, and dermatologists around the world to contribute to their textbooks.

I have strived to make this text relevant for today, with an eye towards what I think is the future of aesthetic medicine, to add the most value for my readers. Our industry is more fast-paced and exciting now than at any time in my career. We are witnessing so many dynamic trends, new technologies, and a plethora of innovative products and practices emerging at record speed which will surely keep us on our toes.

I feel very fortunate to have had the pleasure of being so active in this industry for over two decades and counting. There is much more for me to learn and do; I'm just getting started!

Thank you for reading, and feel free to reach out anytime.

Cheers from New York!
Wendy Lewis
wl@wendylewisco.com
LinkedIn @wendylewisco
LinkedIn Group @globalaestheticprofessionals
Instagram @wendylewisco
Facebook @wendylewiscoltd
X (Twitter) @wendylewisco

About the Author

Wendy Lewis is the Founder and President, since 1997 of Wendy Lewis & Co Ltd. Global Aesthetics Consultancy, a strategic marketing communications group in New York City specializing in the beauty, wellness, and aesthetics categories.

Her group's diverse roster of clients includes healthcare, skincare, medical and energy-based devices, dermatologic brands, start-ups, as well as select aesthetic practices and medspas.

A prolific writer, this marks Lewis's tenth book in publication to date. She is also a prolific writer of articles, features, series, and blogs for numerous publications. Lewis was the recipient of the prestigious *Johnson & Johnson Best Trade Beauty Journalist* award in 2017 and currently serves on the editorial board of *Prime International Anti-Ageing Journal*. She regularly contributes to many prestigious medical journals, including *Aesthetic Society News*, *Modern Aesthetics*, *Practical Dermatology*, *PFMA Journal*, *Aesthetics Journal*, and many other publications and websites.

Wendy is a frequent speaker, course instructor, moderator, and presenter at conferences, webinars, and panels in the US and globally. She serves as an advisor to the Scientific Committee of the FACE Conference & Exhibition in the UK, and on the board of the Aesthetic Tech Forum from Octane.

She is also the founder of the popular LinkedIn group, "Global Aesthetics Professionals," which has over 8,000 members at the time of this printing.

Wendy lives in New York City.

Other Publications from Wendy Lewis

Books

- *Aesthetic Practice Marketing in the Digital Age, First Edition*
- *Practice Makes Perfect: The Complete Cosmetic Beauty Guide*
- *The Beauty Battle: An Insider's Guide*
- *Beauty Secrets: An Insider's Guide to the Latest Skin, Hair & Body Treatments*
- *Complexion Perfection*
- *Wrinkle Rescue*
- *Hair Affair*
- *Figure It Out*
- *The Lowdown on Facelifts and Other Wrinkle Remedies*

Textbook Chapters

- Physician Selection, in Wilkinson TL, ed., *Atlas of Liposuction*, WB Saunders, Philadelphia, 2005.
- The Practice: Models, Management, and Marketing, in Nahai F, ed., *The Art of Aesthetic Surgery: Principles & Techniques*, second edition, Thieme, New York, 2010.
- Fundamentals of Managing and Marketing a Cosmetic Dermatology Clinic in the Modern World, in Andre P, Haneke E, Marini L, Rowland Payne C, eds, *Cosmetic Medicine and Surgery*, CRC Press, Boca Raton 2016, 779-88.
- Managing Your Online Reputation, in Dover JS, Mariwalla, eds, *The Business of Dermatology*, Thieme, New York, 2020.
- Digital Marketing and Social Media Branding, in Sachdev M, Khunger N, eds, *Essentials for Aesthetic Dermatology in Ethnic Skin: Practice and Procedure*, CRC Press, Boca Raton 2023, 243-6.
- High-Yield Business Tips for Dermatologists, in Namazi MR, ed., *Textbook of Dermatological Pearls*, Bentham Science, UAE, forthcoming 2023.

Introduction
Evolution of the Aesthetic Market

Evolution is all about looking forward.

Gerard Piqué Bernabeu, former Spanish professional footballer

The Post-Pandemic Practice

The pandemic caused a dramatic shift in many human behaviors, and it has turned everyday tasks into a minefield of possible viral exposure. Consider the doorknob, for example. What was once a completely innocuous object is now a potential harbinger of deadly disease.

Virtually every hard surface we touch has some potential to carry and transmit the virus. Knowing this, companies are scrambling to find ways to retrofit offices to reduce the number of surfaces employees touch throughout any given workday. Voice technology has a huge role to play in redesigning office spaces so employees can feel safe returning to work.

Shared devices in offices – think computers and monitors, conference call speakers, and projectors – can be upgraded to voice-assisted models which continue to enable collaboration while simultaneously reducing the amount of equipment multiple people touch in a shared space. Contactless keycards, facial recognition, and voice recognition also will likely form at least part of the building security picture in the near-term and post-pandemic workplace. Yet, aesthetic practices are still finding it difficult to hire staff, including medical professionals and administrative staff.

Many senior dermatologists, plastic surgeons, and facial plastic surgeons are considering all their options. To sell or not to sell is a common debate across the specialty. Some of my colleagues are concerned that if they don't join a big group now, they may miss out on the best opportunities, while others are debating the prospect of having a boss after being in solo practice for most of their careers. There are also looming concerns surrounding the competition coming from the medspa market, which is stimulating more interest in reconsidering all options. Staffing continues to be a big challenge for all practitioners as today's employees are less likely to be loyal to employers and have set the bar quite high to stay long term. Turnover of key staff members can have a significant impact on practices in terms of the loss of institutional memory, the inherent costs of training, and the stress it puts on the staff and practitioners.

There was a time when it was widely accepted that aesthetic patients would only go to board-certified dermatologists or plastic surgeons for minimally invasive treatments. However, the post-pandemic state of aesthetics has altered that perception in the minds of many patients who are keen to take advantage of the benefits offered by medspa chains, including memberships and subscriptions, affordable pricing, flexible scheduling, and other user-friendly options.

Aesthetics Goes Mainstream

The landscape of aesthetic patients has been expanding in recent years, perhaps despite a global pandemic and/or because of it.

We are seeing new categories of patients of all age groups who are starting to have treatments earlier. This trend has fostered a plethora of new clinic models sprouting up in all markets including medspa chains, group practices, dermatology centers, and more recently, even plastic surgery practices have morphed from the traditional solo practice model to joining groups.

Solo practices are becoming cost-prohibitive to operate in many markets and some practitioners may find it harder to compete with large groups and centers. More multi-specialty centers are popping up as a "one-stop shopping" experience for aesthetic patients.

During the early days of COVID in New York, when most purely aesthetic practices were on lockdown for several months, there were many homes in the Hamptons that opened their doors to a few A-list physicians who came to treat a group of eager patients for BOTOX® and other essentials under the radar. That trend has stuck in many markets now. Have syringe, will travel…

WHAT DO AESTHETIC PATIENTS WANT?

For starters, they want convenience in terms of easy access to treatments and products, same-day and next-day availability, ease of scheduling remotely, virtual consultations and follow-ups, curbside pickup for product purchases, service menus that include a wide range of options, loyalty programs, memberships, and subscription models. Aesthetic patients are less impressed with credentials like an Ivy League education and a prestigious residency and are more interested in practitioners' Instagram and TikTok channels, which is where many of them are finding the clinics they go to.

Increased Innovation

Aesthetic surgery and non-invasive treatments are on the uptick as consumer interest has grown over the past few years, despite the global pandemic. We are seeing more and more practitioners, from physicians to nurses and other specialists in different markets, dipping a toe into the lucrative aesthetic treatment category that, by all accounts, has proven to be recession-proof.

More people are investigating procedures across the spectrum from surgical to minimally invasive. This trend has encouraged more consumer groups to enter the market earlier from Gen Z to millennials. There has also been a growing demand for aesthetic treatments for men of all ages, most notably injectable treatments, hair restoration, rhinoplasty, as well as non-invasive body shaping.

This dovetails with the advancements in the industry that continue to experience an influx of new technologies which have made treatments and procedures faster, less uncomfortable and invasive, and safer for doctors to delegate to ancillary staff. Advances in laser technology, for example, continue to make procedures faster, more efficient, less painful, and more effective. The use of robotics in surgery is also expected to become more common.

As the industry expands its services, with more people taking advantage of minimally invasive procedures, the market for non-surgical treatments is expected to grow significantly in the coming years due to their affordability, convenience, and wide acceptance globally.

In the future, the industry is likely to focus on refining existing procedures and treatments to ensure a very high level of safety. There has been an increased focus on novel, minimally invasive technologies, such as lasers and radiofrequency treatments, and injectables for the face as well as the body.

The medical aesthetics sector presents appealing opportunities for investors and private equity funds. Three major factors are behind that strong outlook:

1. A huge untapped potential among consumers.
2. Significant investments from both private equity funds and manufacturers.
3. Track records of fast recovery from previous economic dips.

Mergers and Acquisitions

The dermatology and medical aesthetics markets continue to grow and expand in many parts of the world, not just in the US. These popular specialties seem to be practically recession-proof as they have weathered the market fluctuations and continue to attract a wide range of investors, plus a plethora of patients who continue to enter the market.

The multi-billion dollar, global dermatology and aesthetics markets continue to thrive and evolve, and there is strong interest among many newcomers entering the market from consumer products, dentistry, and other new segments.

Post-Pandemic Perceptions

The characteristic "lipstick effect" awakened consumers to advanced beauty experiences for pampering and calming. Aesthetic treatments and products have a soothing effect that makes patients feel more relaxed. From self-care facials and body treatments to injectables, lasers, and light-based therapies, the global medical aesthetics industry has held its own during the pandemic and beyond.

The aesthetics market seems to have rallied even faster than expected. The steady recovery has created a plethora of patients who are eager to get back to their treatment regimens and invest even more time and funds to new and new-ish treatments, allowing many practices to experience steady, post-pandemic growth.

Most aesthetic practices bounced back relatively quickly from the pandemic, and many were able to rebound in a healthier and happier state. Undoubtedly, the way you practice and manage patients has changed. While none of us would have chosen a global pandemic as a defining event in our lives, the bright side is that we learned some hard lessons that will serve us well for years to come.

For example, more practitioners have readily embraced non-surgical treatments as a highly lucrative addition to their practices. Professional skin care sales carried many practices through the lockdown by implementing drop shipping, curbside pickup, Shopify, and Facebook/Instagram stores. Practitioners who were initially resistant to the concept of telemedicine, virtual consults, follow-ups, and events, have now embraced these trends with open arms and are fully onboard.

There is also a realization that you may not really need a cavernous waiting room anymore and prefer not having patients and their friends and family present for consults and procedures. To that end, many practices re-engineered their space to get the best return on pricey square footage.

Some of us have emerged with stronger management skills, a healthier respect for the bottom line, and a desire for leaner and more efficient systems. The pandemic changed our thinking and left us with the time to automate many day-to-day tasks and change the way we practice to prioritize efficiency. We have sold, donated, or traded up capital equipment, and eliminated a lot of waste in our businesses.

The mainstream adoption of working from home has impacted the workforce in the long term. Considering the undeniable benefits of the remote workforce, many companies have adopted some form of work-from-home model, at least for staff who do not have direct client contact, including bookkeepers, accountants, schedulers, administrative staff, marketing and social media support, and computer techs.

Faced with a shortage of qualified staff, keeping your best people happy translates to lower turnover and loss of institutional memory. The concept of "work-life balance" which once seemed like a myth to many of us, has taken on new meaning. Being able to spend more time with your kids, take a yoga class, or meet a colleague for coffee certainly has its advantages.

1

Modern Aesthetic Patient Experience

Never lose sight of the fact that the most important yardstick of your success will be how you treat other people.

Barbara Bush, First Lady of the United States

High-Tech Clinics Emerging

Undoubtedly, the future of all fields lies in technological advancements that enable greater efficiency and cost savings. Insurance companies, hospitals, governmental regulations, and investors are driving this trend. Even in the case of elective procedures, these changes have a knock-on effect on how aesthetic practices operate.

We have been forced to embrace technology. In some cases, we did it by kicking and screaming (you know who you are). This has left some old-school physicians to wonder whether the traditional, deeply personal doctor-patient connection is becoming a thing of the past.

One of the many benefits of investing in technology is that it provides data that helps to facilitate educated decisions for your business. The analytics you get from Google, social media management platforms, and practice management software are valuable tools and insights that may impact everything from clinical decisions, documentation, treatment plans, forecasting business growth, and determining how best to utilize your marketing budget and staff.

A decade or so ago, it was very challenging for a new practitioner to become established in a market where mature practices held a grip on the upper echelon of patients. However, more recently, with the advent of social media and digital marketing, an ambitious physician who is social media savvy can rise to global stardom with a limited budget in record time.

The Virtual Practice

Consider offering online scheduling of virtual consults.

If your staff is conducting consultations through Zoom or Microsoft Teams, have written rules in place. For example, if you don't allow your medical staff to prescribe certain medications in person, make sure that rule carries over to virtual consults.

Another way to take advantage of the 'virtual' trend is to offer gift cards, memberships, and other models directly through your website so patients can tap into the services and products you offer online. Check your local regulations before using this model as rules will differ from market to market.

Offering gift cards via the practice website provides clients flexibility to use them for any service or product they want in the practice in terms of products or services with no expiration.

Demise of the Solo Practitioner

Solo practice is a concept that has a very short lifespan in the current state of medicine in general. The costs of running a thriving practice are too high for a single physician to bear the entire burden,

DOI: 10.1201/9780429356742-1

especially if they are in the early days of running a practice. It is not a scalable model when you factor in all the expenses needed to open a clinic and thrive. For example, a laser can cost upwards of $250,000 US, malpractice insurance is a hefty expense, and a substantial marketing budget is essential to attracting patients and driving revenue.

Many solo practices across specialties are selling out to private equity-backed chains and medical centers or joining groups. Thus, group practices are flourishing, which offers new opportunities for physicians and physician extenders to practice their craft without having to shell out the excruciating overhead costs.

The Art of Empathy

The pandemic changed how we market and catapulted us into a digital transformation perhaps sooner than expected. The sudden shift in consumer behavior caused everyone to adapt quickly to a new model. Those who were slow to adapt found their practices lagging behind the competition. This period made it clear that your marketing approach should be more customer-focused than ever before.

Zoom and other platforms that facilitate virtual consults and meetings with patients have had a huge impact on the aesthetics industry. The over-hyped phenomenon coined as "Zoom dysmorphia" has stuck post-pandemic. Overall, there was an increase in appointments for appearance-related issues, perhaps most notably in appointments related to rhinoplasty and injectables to treat the upper face, and "tech neck," which refers to the lower face and jowls.

Patients need multiple touchpoints, including some nurturing, reassurance, and convincing before they sign up, especially for invasive procedures. This is even more germane among an older population of patients who may be more concerned with their health.

To remain competitive, outstanding digital content is a critical success factor for getting consumers to engage, building connections with your audience, and retaining their interest in your practice for when they are ready to have surgery, a treatment, or purchase skincare. The traditional methods of acquiring new patients have stopped working as well, or at all anymore, so practices need to pivot quickly. Converting live events, patient visits, and consultations to virtual options is helping many practices thrive. Many of the alternative strategies that were adopted have lasted post-pandemic because they were efficient, cost-effective, and both patients and practitioners got used to practicing this way.

The most effective way to reach new clients who may become loyal patients is to take a patient-centric approach. This approach entails talking less, listening more, and being more sensitive to patients' needs. While some aesthetic clients may appear to have a short attention span and think they know what they want and need, kindness goes a long way in building relationships. They will remember how you made them feel.

Connecting with Patients

New technologies emerged to improve our methods of communication. Everything digital took center stage as we relied on our devices to connect and socialize. With social distancing, human connections became increasingly important, especially for customer service. Smarter technology allowed brands to adapt quickly and anticipate the changing needs of consumers.

These changes will be long-lasting and continue to evolve at a rapid pace. Most consumers did not go back to baseline post-pandemic practices. In fact, we continue to rely on digital technologies as they arise and get easier to use.

The willingness to implement new business practices and communication is not a trend. Leveraging digital technologies and embracing the shifts has allowed businesses to stay efficient, lean, mean, and flourish. One of the keys to success is to stay engaged with the topics that matter most to your audience, and to join those conversations in a valuable and impactful way. Consumers will always crave a human connection.

**5 Steps to Navigate the
Patient/Client Journey**

1. Develop a connection
2. Understand their goals, concerns, pain
   points
3. Address key wants & needs
4. Define a plan with solutions &
   alternatives
5. Maintain a long-term relationship
   through trust

Revisiting the Aesthetic Consultation

The consultation process has changed with the impact of technology. Virtual consultations have become standard operating procedure. My GP at Mount Sinai Hospital in New York offers the option of virtual consults for everything but your annual physical. Forms are completed online in advance, fees are pre-paid via credit card, and the visits are scheduled for 30-minute slots, which is a huge time-saver for both the doctor and the patient.

Many cosmetic patients appreciate the convenience of not having to travel for an initial consultation. Failing to offer the option of consultations via Zoom, Microsoft Teams, or another platform of choice may prove to be a barrier to attracting some patients, especially for those who live a long distance away. Virtual consults, follow-ups, and events have become standard operating procedure in many practices.

Video consultations can cut down on lead times for an appointment, reduce patient travel pre- and post-procedure, and allow other specialists and staff members to be online with the patient. This can be a win-win so everyone is happy.

Modern aesthetic practices utilize an intake form on an iPad for patients while they wait, so their information is automatically entered into the system seamlessly. Other advances involve digital photography, which is far ahead of the curve. The technology is more compact and simplified, yet results may be more accurate. Relying on software, rather than expensive equipment that takes up valuable space, ticks another box for streamlining your practice.

Innovative technology helps make our day-to-day lives more efficient, thus we continue to embrace automation to increase efficiency, and reduce time, costs, and unnecessary stress.

The Non-Waiting Room

Whereas formerly the waiting room and front desk were the lifelines of every practice, in the new world order, these areas may be reconfigured or repurposed. If you practice in a crowded metropolitan area where real estate is at a premium, a patient waiting area may be the first thing to go. Poorly utilized or non-essential space can be converted to add an extra treatment room with a wall or partition. This strategy goes straight to your bottom line.

Having patients check in via text or phone when their rooms were ready worked well in locations where patients could wait in their air-conditioned minivans. In New York or London, they may have had to stand outside in the cold or rain or scramble to find the nearest Starbucks. Patients are busy too, and they don't like to be kept waiting, so these alternatives proved to be keepers for many practices.

Skincare and other products and testers may be moved out of waiting rooms and relocated to treatment rooms. Practices and medspas may offer curbside pickup and shipping for product sales and replenishment for convenience. Pre-selling patients before their appointment proved to be an efficient strategy. Virtual consults and events helped facilitate that model that has become the new normal in many practices.

Many practitioners and business owners have had a sea change in their whole way of thinking. We tend to be more concerned about the environment, and at least some of us emerged to be just a little bit kinder to each other and more inclined to value the people around us, including family, friends, colleagues, and patients.

It took a global health crisis for us to change our way of doing business and to treat each other with more compassion. I see this as a very positive change.

> *Save a Tree! Glossy brochures, fancy folders, before and after instructions, and other collateral materials that were once displayed in patient areas are obsolete now. These have been replaced by digital alternatives, such as a monitor with a looped reel of the key treatments offered or a YouTube channel with robust educational videos. Pre- and post-procedure instructions can be shared electronically. Prescriptions are now submitted seamlessly to the patient's pharmacy. Appointments can be confirmed or rescheduled via text messaging, etc. Dealing with paperwork and being stuck on hold is just a time suck.*

Streamlining Your Business

Some may say that purging your office of stuff you don't want or need is better than sex. I would tend to agree.

Decluttering can be a very cathartic experience. Post-pandemic, many practices dumped their clipboards and waved farewell to glossy handouts. Patient forms are now digitized and updated frequently to stay current, including pre- and post-procedure instructions, consents, fee quotes, intake forms, etc. Including a password-protected Patient Portal on your website also increases efficiency as patients can access the forms and information they need at any time by using their personal code.

Another task on your to-do list is to take a deep dive into what is happening (or not happening) in the treatment rooms. Those who are hanging on to antiquated technology, like an oversized facial machine or skincare products patients are not buying, have a reason to get rid of it.

Evaluate all your expenses and cut corners on anything that is non-essential, does not impact the patient experience, or does not make money for the business. Vendors may be more understanding, and even extend their payment terms. Look for ways to cut expenses to improve your bottom line.

Anything that doesn't generate revenue or added value to the practice has hopefully been given away or abandoned. Investing in high-efficacy products and branded services that patients are looking for serves to elevate your practice and the bottom line.

Consumer expectations and perspectives have shifted. The patient experience has changed from how we knew it, which has led the way to more creative thinking towards building authentic connections with patients. We also learned that we need a lot less stuff to bog us down in all aspects of our lives. So, keep your practice nimble, efficient, and updated to focus on what really matters: taking exceptional care of patients and clients, delivering superior outcomes, offering the products and services that your patients want, keeping staff happy to minimize turnover, and avoiding burnout.

Six Strategies for Success

1. Carefully monitor the customer journey for improvements 24/7.
2. Create a plan to respond in real time on all the channels your patients are active on.
3. Continually test new and improved methods of reaching your target audience.
4. Reward longtime patients and staff for their loyalty.
5. Create original content that only "members" can view to make them feel special and a part of your exclusive group.
6. Show gratitude to your team for everything they do for you and your business.

PATH TO PATIENT LOYALTY

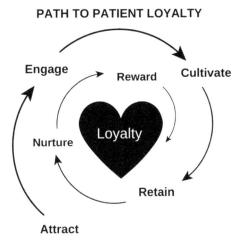

Lessons Learned

Be responsive today and proactive for tomorrow.

Protect your business, assets, and facility from whatever threat may be coming next – and there will be one because there always is. Hang on to the staff who really matter to your business by taking good care of them and letting them know you appreciate everything they do for your business and patients.

Don't leave yourself unprepared and vulnerable for when the next disaster hits.

2

Business of Branding and Rebranding

Your brand is what other people say about you when you're not in the room.

Jeff Bezos, Founder of Amazon

What should come first, marketing or branding?

That is akin to asking the age-old question, "chicken vs. egg." You need a chicken to make an egg, and you need marketing to promote your brand.

It is a natural mistake to confuse marketing with branding, yet there is a distinct difference between these two essential methods of self-promotion.

The main goal of marketing is to make your business look so great to people, that it piques the audience's interest you can convert them to become paying customers. This usually means spending a fair amount of time what your market really wants.

The next step is to consider the best ways of connecting your products and services with what your target audience is looking for. Once you have gone through this exercise you will be equipped to spread the word about how your products and services are in sync with what your target audience wants and needs.

The Rationale for Branding

When marketing messages are unclear about what your brand stands for, you may fall into the trap of trying to become who or what the market wants you to be, rather than who you truly are. This strategy is certain to fail because it undermines the important elements of trust and transparency for your brand. Thus, branding and marketing may play equal roles in promoting your products and services to the market, but they come at it from slightly different angles.

The task of branding is to consistently support who you are and how you are perceived by all the stakeholders that matter. Everyone must be in lockstep with the core culture, mission, messaging, and "raison d'être" of your business. A successful brand should be instantly meaningful to anyone who encounters it. It may be the most important deciding factor for consumers when they make a purchasing decision. It gives your practice an identity beyond just the products or services you offer that can be found in many or most aesthetic practices.

This doesn't happen overnight. Can you have one without the other? The short answer is yes, but the wiser answer is no way!

Investing in marketing your practice without first nailing down what you want your brand to stand for is taking a shortcut that won't serve you well over time. Branding your practice will give you the advantage you need to stand out in the ever-expanding crowd of aesthetic practices and medspas. It will also make you more relatable to the target audience of consumers that you want to attract.

Defining Your Brand

From the color palette of your website, the tone of your Instagram posts, the look and feel of the products and services you offer, and the entire staff in the clinic, everything you do factors into how your brand is perceived my patients, colleagues, and the media. A brand's name is more than a label or a logo; it should evoke a feeling that translates to customer expectations.

DOI: 10.1201/9780429356742-2

Your brand creates connectivity and loyalty with customers and patients. It delivers an emotional and loyal bond with each of them that translates to customer loyalty, growth, and profits.

Strong brands tend to appeal to the widest net of customers, which means those brands are more likely to be chosen before their competitors. Branding your practice in the right way will help you stand out from the crowd so you will be preferred and remembered by the target audience you want to attract.

Your brand can be one of your most important assets if it encourages more patients to seek you out and buy from you. An added benefit is that the whole staff may be more loyal when they are proud of the brand they represent, and it will be easier to recruit additional staff and partners.

Think of your brand as a living entity that is either enriched or undermined cumulatively over time by every choice you make, no matter how small.

What Adjectives Best Describe Who You Are as a Practitioner?

Think about how you want to be perceived. Then consider the key messages you want to convey to patients or clients.

For example, your brand may stand for "high-quality service" and "cutting-edge treatments." However, those terms tend to define what you do rather than who you are as a practitioner.

Do you want to be known as an expert who is well-trained, highly experienced, and has superb technique? Or would you prefer to be thought of as approachable, having a good bedside manner, and very caring?

These choices are different, but not mutually exclusive.

FIVE QUESTIONS TO CONSIDER WHEN BUILDING YOUR BRAND

1. *What is your primary target audience?*
2. *What is your secondary target audience?*
3. *Who are you most eager to connect with?*
4. *How do you want prospective patients to think of you?*
5. *How would you like your peers to think of you?*

The tone and voice of your communications, including emails, social media, adverts, website, plus office location, and décor set the stage. Patients will often decide whether they trust you to treat them from their very first encounter, which might be on Instagram or TikTok, or just by walking past your business.

The way you think about your patient relationships should be in sync with how you think about your brand. What do you tell your patients during a consultation to make them trust you as a person as well as a professional?

Your branding touchpoints include your online presence, physical presence, print collateral, waiting room, staff uniforms, and every form of communication that touches your current patients as well at prefered target audience.

Eight Steps to Distinguish Your Brand and Stay Relevant

1. Determine your primary and secondary target audiences, for example, this may be women over 40 seeking out anti-aging treatments plus millennials looking for acne treatments and 'Baby Botox".
2. Establish how you want to be perceived by patients, colleagues, vendors, local businesses, etc. These may be slightly different for each group, but it should be consistent in terms of quality and style.
3. Define your core values, features, and benefits, who are you as a medical professional?

4. Create your visual assets, logo, color pallette, look and feel, design, etc.
5. Identify your brand voice and tone.
6. Put your branding to work to elevate your practice so it stands out in the marketplace.
7. Maintain and protect your brand with a vengeance!
8. Rebrand when it is no longer working, or your business has moved on to the next level.

Your primary target audience may be "new patients" generally, but the specific demographic may vary considerably. For example, you may be eager to attract more women over 40 because that group tends to be very motivated to have aesthetic treatments and is often in a good position with the funds and/or credit to invest.

Millennials, or Gen Y, are another group that represents a growing number of aesthetic patients. This group has proven to be a universally important demographic for medical aesthetics in most markets.

Male patients are steadily on the rise for aesthetic treatments, from injectables, hair restoration, laser resurfacing and body sculpting. Overlook this demographic at your own peril!

In most metropolitan areas, men and millennials are now well-established as highly engaged patient groups. To ensure that your brand resonates with them, consider their age, location, interests, professions, and lifestyle, as well as their unique personality traits.

Your target audiences may be approachable through the social media channels they spend the most time on industry partners, colleagues, and friends.

This is a useful exercise to analyze your patient population and make sure you are catering to their specific needs and goals.

Defining Your Practice or Medspa Brand

Your business brand is a lot more than just a logo, a tagline, and a color scheme. Your brand is a crucial asset that will help shape a positive perception of your business in the minds of consumers, peers, neighbors, industry colleagues, and the media.

If you get it right and stay true to your brand's principles for the long term, they will become aware of who you are and what you stand for. This can crystallize your practice's key values, personality, mission, and positioning. If you fail at this important exercise by straying from your brand's principles, you will be undermining all the hard work you and your staff have invested in.

Striving to build a strong brand has numerous advantages in the uber-competitive aesthetic medicine market. For example, a strong brand builds enhanced recognition, patient loyalty, increased value to your target audience, credibility, and overall trust. A strong brand will help to generate awareness, word of mouth recommendations, and help your practice stand out from the competition. In turn, this means you can attract new leads and convert them into long-term patients, considering people who share your values and mission are more likely to be interested in what you have to offer.

Another important benefit of building a brand, rather than just another practice, is to attract a dynamic team of like-minded individuals who will be on board with your mission and goals. A team of rock stars who genuinely support your values and principles will tend to be more loyal and committed. Hopefully, the result is that they will stay with you for the long haul. However, in the crowded aesthetics market, some staff turnover is to be expected. If it becomes too frequent, find out why.

Aesthetic patients today tend to recommend their favorite brands and practitioners to friends and colleagues. They tend to be more likely to share their experiences and mention their doctors and practices by name to friends and their social media fans and followers. Word of mouth is critically important to spread the word about your clinic or medspa.

Patients and clients who are indifferent towards the brand they have a relationship with present a window of opportunity to be converted come to your practice. This may be accomplished by offering something they have not found elsewhere, such as state-of-the-art treatments, exquisitely well-trained staff, up-to-the-minute treatments and products, or a uniquely high-end experience.

Caveat: The biggest mistake you can make is to do nothing and simply wait for patients to come to you. Get proactive and develop a business plan stat!

Keep It Simple Stupid

One of the pillars of brand building is the basic concept of simplicity. An important strategy for developing a brand is distilling what you want to say down to a word or two, an experience, or a feeling.

Think about some of the brands you really admire.

EMFACE® BY BTL

This is a very popular and pricey facial tightening technology. What do consumers think when they see that brand name? Some words that may come to mind are "innovative," "trending," "bold," and "high-tech." The brand's marketing speaks to these qualities, and they have invested heavily in celebrities, sports figures, charities, and special events to drive their key messages home to prospective patients. BTL has mastered the challenge of keeping their brand top of mind.

We often come across brands that lose out by trying to be everything to everyone. Avoid this trap by drafting a straightforward message that is specific, ownable, and memorable. You should be able to explain your brand in as few words as possible so it will be readily understood. Simple and distinctive messaging is more likely to connect with your audience and stay top of mind. Try to avoid names and phrases that are hard to remember, tricky to spell, or challenging to pronounce.

If you want patients to truly connect with your brand, they should be nurtured to experience a positive reaction when they see your logo and read about your practice. This can help to create an emotional experience that tends to keep patients coming back and sending their friends.

Invest in your brand as early as possible in the evolution of your practice. Always aim to do better while maintaining the important pillars of your brand so patients and clients will know what to expect. Once you have created a strong message and image, it will naturally evolve over time as your brand continues to grow and expand.

Authenticity is an important component of effective brand building. Without that element, your brand will suffer from being unpredictable, which is the opposite of what you want to convey.

Aesthetic patients don't like surprises; they want to know what to expect every time they come to see you. Your brand should pull together every aspect of your practice so you can communicate this ethos clearly and reinforce it 365 days a year.

Brand Building vs. Brand Breaking

One of the caveats of brand building is simplicity. This important component of developing a brand distills what you want to say down to a few words, an experience, or a feeling. Some brands lose out by trying to be everything to everyone by drafting a complicated message that is neither ownable nor memorable. You should be able to explain your own brand in as few words as possible so it can be readily understood.

To build a brand that will serve you over time, choose a straightforward and clear message that can resonate with your target audience. Brands that aren't memorable or sound too much like other brands so they are not distinquistable are destined to be 'brand breakers'.

Your marketing should consistently help to create a familiar emotional experience which tends to keep patients coming back. They should be made to feel positive when they see your logo and marketing. Any change in tone is not on brand sends a message to patients that they may not have the same experience every time they come in. To protect your brand, communicate its ethos clearly and reinforce it in everything you say and do.

Protecting Your Brand

Branding will serve to support your marketing and advertising plan and help to boost promotional activities through added recognition and impact. Keep your brand strong by diligently maintaining every detail. This includes managing the basic elements of your brand (style guide, packaging, color palette, treatment menu, service, etc.), as well as how your brand is perceived by your audience and customer base.

Caveat: Before you make any major decisions, ask yourself, "Is this on brand for us?" If you have to think hard about it to decide, it probably isn't.

Think of your brand as a living, breathing asset that needs to be maintained for the long term. Do you deliver on your marketing promises? Do you and your staff go above and beyond to live up to what the brand conveys to patients?

Strong branding builds trust with clients, patients, and partners. If you let patients down by easing up on maintaining the principles protecting your brand, you may risk losing their trust which may be hard or impossible to get back.

Create a consistent image so followers can easily recognize your brand when you post content and when they see your promotions or ads. Your company logo is the first visual representation people will see of your brand. Make sure that you are using a recognizable brand image (your logo) so followers can easily recognize your brand when you post content.

Measuring the worth or value of a brand is qualitative, not quantitative. There will be quantitative offshoots, but if what you are putting out is true to your brand, you can be successful.

Always think about how you can improve your brand. Building a high-quality evergreen brand doesn't happen overnight. It takes years of due diligence to get there, but the rewards will be well worth it.

HOW DO YOU KNOW WHEN IT'S TIME FOR A REBRAND?

- *Is your brand outdated by today's standards?*
- *Are you still clinging to the logo you started with a few decades ago?*
- *Is your "color" palette black and white?*
- *Is "Times New Roman" your font of choice?*
- *When was the last time you checked your whole website?*
- *Do your business cards just have your office phone number?*

These and other signs are practically flashing at you in boldface: **REBRAND ME!**

The Process of Rebranding

Brands – just like fashion, logos, color palettes, and fonts – tend to come and go out of style. Remember when peach was a popular paint palette for plastic surgery practices because it was deemed to be feminine, and silk flowers were fashionable in the waiting room? Unfortunately, I do.

Your brand is much more than just a logo. It reflects who you are as a professional and is both tangible and intangible. Just like your own identity, your brand is always evolving.

Rebranding is not just about a new logo or website with all the bells and whistles. It's about the entire look and feel of your brand which is reflected to the world. To maintain continuity, the new image should be complementary rather than dramatically different or unrecognizable, which risks a loss of brand equity.

Eight Reasons Why You Need a Rebrand

1. Your company has evolved beyond its previous identity.
2. The brand has become outdated.
3. The brand's aesthetics no longer match your core values.
4. You are branching out into new territories: products, location, business model, and partners.
5. The key target demographic has changed over time.
6. The competitive landscape has changed.
7. You're ready to take your brand to the next level.
8. Your practice has taken on a new partner.

Conduct frequent checks on your branding to assess whether it still feels modern and current and relays the right messages.

If you want to come across as innovative, forward-thinking, and up on trends in modern aesthetics, your branding needs to reflect those traits. Rebranding provides an opportunity to strengthen your brand's presence and image in the eyes of your clients while maintaining the elements that make you stand apart.

Price vs. Value

Price is simply what something costs; it's strictly a numbers game and quantitative. But value is more emotional. Value can be defined as the worth or importance people assign to a product, thing, experience, or person. It considers the usefulness and benefits that mean different things to different people.

Commoditization is all about price comparison. Unfortunately, we see a lot of this tactic in medical aesthetics, especially as a major component of big chain business models. High traffic and low prices often translate to higher marketing spending to continually bring in new patients. This can be a losing battle because someone is always willing to do it or sell it for less. The most valuable patients you want to attract tend to have very little loyalty to practices that operate like this.

Consider there is a sunk cost to every treatment or procedure in an aesthetics practice. This may range from the cost of the device, any consumable required, staff time involved, typing up a treatment room, as well as the cost per acquisition of a customer. Practices that rely on a low price to get patients in the door rarely have high retention rates. The patients they attract are not sticky; they tend to always be looking for the next best deal. They rarely convert into loyal patients who will stick with you for the long term.

Strategies to Keep Patients Coming Back

Face facts. Aesthetic patients have a lot of choices today, and they know how to leverage that power.

They are being courted by a wide range of your competitors. They look to some media outlets, share notes with their friends and family, and post about their experiences online.

Undoubtedly, more patients of all age groups and income levels are eager to take advantage of perks, especially from the medspas and clinic chains leading the way. Consumers are programmed to shop around for the best providers, fair prices, aftercare, location, and price point, especially Gen X and Gen Y.

In this crowded market, many aesthetics practices are taking the lead from retailers, airlines, hotel chains, and Amazon for fresh ways to attract new patients and keep them coming back without straying. Well-constructed programs can increase customer retention rates by keeping them engaged with your practice. It can also be a cost-effective way to acquire new patients and lure patients who have strayed to come back.

Patient Perks, Plans, and Promos

These perks and plans can be structured in many ways to align with your goals and patient demographic.

- Leverage exclusive content, first access to new products, favorable pricing, quarterly bundles, and more.
- Upsell frequent fliers to sign on for special programs and offers that you feature.
- Allow patients to access a plan that can be customized just for them and include a select array of treatments – for example, fillers, toxins, and facial treatments.

Loyalty programs: Keep patients coming back by enlisting them in an ongoing loyalty program, starting from the first treatment they have or the first product they buy. They can collect points with every treatment that entitles them to additional benefits in your practice and encourages them to stay with you. A "friends and family" concept can also fit into this program model.

Subscription services: For repetitive treatments, consider creating a subscription plan that offers the best prices on multiple treatment categories and products. One popular strategy is to present a well-structured subscription model to first-time treatment patients that ticks all the boxes to keep them on board. Add another other valuable perk exclusively for frequent buyers over time.

Memberships: Memberships create natural customer touchpoints including semi-annual offers, holiday gifts, product samples, special events, and sneak peeks at new products and treatments. You may start by enrolling patients who make a purchase to the membership program or create your own model that works best for your practice.

Tiered pricing: Many practices offer different fees based on tiers or the number of treatments the patient has purchased. The more they buy, the lower the tier price becomes. Consider pricing the first treatment at the going rate in your market, then add 15 to 20% off for a second and third treatment as an example. You may also set a price for a tier and discount the second tier for the patient.

Add More Value to Treatments

Don't just lower your prices!

Lowering your fees can send the wrong message – such as you are desperate for new patients or you're not very busy. Change your way of thinking to stifle any potential impulse to start discounting.

Instead of slashing your fees, try offering something extra to add value to the treatments you offer. Best practice is to introduce clients to something new that they have not experienced yet.

Bundling treatments: Consider bundling or mix-and-match packages, such as a toxin treatment with a laser hair removal package for select patients or adding radiofrequency (RF) to a mommy makeover procedure. This is a way to introduce the patient to another treatment they may not have experienced before.

Special perks: To show appreciation to a loyal patient who has sent referrals, gift them with complimentary treatment in a series they are having to show your appreciation. This strategy may also serve as a goodwill gesture to convert a patient who is not entirely happy to become an advocate. This strategy also dissuade a client from posting a negative review online.

Gift with purchase (GWP): Give this tried and true tactic – credited to Estée Lauder – a facelift. Get creative by using this model with a twist, by offering enhanced value to the client.

- Choose a time frame that is easy for patients to access in-person or virtually, such as after 5:00 PM or lunchtime. Try a "buy one – get one" theme to move products that are not selling well or of which you have a lot of inventory. This model could offer two of the same product, the same brand/different product, or a product plus travel size.

- Design a "buy one for (set a minimum price) – get a complimentary full-sized product as our gift." It could be from the same brand or a different brand and set a maximum value for the gift product. Try this pre-holidays or at a meaningful date for your practice, like your tenth anniversary, etc.

Need some fresh ideas for loyalty programs and rewards?

Check out the Beauty Insider program from Sephora which is hailed as the best-in-class program on offer.

Look for inspiration from airlines, hotels, restaurant chains, coffee chains, and department stores like Saks Fifth Ave, Galleries Lafayette, Harrods, and more.

THE PARETO PRINCIPLE

We have all heard this cliché a million times, but it bears repeating.

"20% of your clients bring in 80% of your business."

And another oldie but goodie to keep in mind:

"20% of your clients are responsible for 80% of your client complaints."

Keeping It Real

In this uber-competitive environment, once a client has made contact, or had a consultation, or a treatment to nurture that relationship.

Building trust helps clients to feel secure and safe in the knowledge that they have found the right clinic with experts at what they do. Strive to always make your patients and clients feel valued and appreciated, or, as we know, they will find a clinic that fulfills those needs. If they like your team and the treatment they receive in your practice, they are much more likely to come back.

TIPS TO STAY COMPETITIVE IN AN EVER-CHANGING LANDSCAPE FROM WEBTOOLS

- *Stay at the top of the pack by implementing tools as they become popular, such as online appointment scheduling and a text messaging system that will let patients communicate with your staff by SMS.*
- *Each month, devote 30 minutes to reading new blog posts featuring how to market cosmetic treatments. Alternatively, appoint a team member who will stay current with new technologies and may also help implement them or find vendors who will.*
- *Identify peers and vendors you can bounce ideas off. Find out what other clinics experience in terms of trends, macroeconomics, new tools, and AI. Ask their opinions on new technologies before you purchase them.*
- *Spot-check email communication with patients and recorded phone calls, to make sure staff members are following your guidelines and scripts. Ask to see reports to measure how effective team members are in converting leads to appointments.*

Source: https://webtoolsgroup.com/

3

Strategic Primer for Digital Marketing

It's important to remember your competitor is only one mouse click away.

Douglas Warner III, Former CEO and Chairman of the Board of J.P. Morgan & Co.

Keeping up with the current climate and trends in digital marketing takes a small army.

Strategies for digital marketing are constantly in flux because it is such a moving target. Having a modern, trending website with all the bells and whistles is still important, but it just isn't enough anymore.

In fact, if you are keen to attract a younger patient population, they probably won't even look at your website and jump right to your Instagram or TikTok to decide if they want to make an appointment.

Whereas many tried and true marketing tactics will stand the test of time, digital marketing trends and tools tend to morph at a rapid pace. Year after year, the tactics that have worked well for you in the past may need to be redesigned or cast aside to keep up with the most up-to-date trends.

Algorithms change on a whim. We are constantly at the mercy of the "Google Gods" to figure out how to increase conversion rates, and who has time for that? I'm guessing that most practitioners would rather be injecting lips or reshaping thighs rather than logging in to a tech forum to get intel about Google.

CRASH COURSE ON DIGITAL MARKETING

Digital marketing uses search engines, social media, websites, phone and tablet apps to connect and engage potential customers.

Six Must-Have Digital Marketing Strategies

1. *Search Engine Optimization (SEO).*
2. *Pay-Per-Click Advertising (PPC).*
3. *Content Marketing to target defined audiences.*
4. *Social Media Marketing (SMM).*
5. *Emails and Text Marketing.*
6. *Online Reputation Management (ORM 9).*

Digital marketing offers the highest return on investment or ROI. It is also the most direct and effective method for lead generation at a reasonable cost based on your goals and with measurable outcomes.

Diversifying your marketing strategies and adopting more digital options is the clear path to success for aesthetic practices and medspas.

The Perennial Power of Digital

To stay competitive and flourish, a comprehensive digital strategy is a critical success factor for aesthetic practices and medspas in the current climate.

DOI: 10.1201/9780429356742-3

Traditional old-school marketing tactics need to be upgraded to stay current and meet patient expectations of today. Printed materials, brochures, forms, and snail mail have long been replaced with text messaging which can put patients in touch with you in a matter of seconds.

Your marketing goals need to be clear, realistic, and aligned with your business objectives from the start. Maintaining consistent messaging, tone, and visuals across all channels is important to stay on brand.

Identify your target audience to focus on the patients you want to attract. This will help guide you to create tailored marketing campaigns to connect with each of these targets. Once you have narrowed down your targets, you can choose the best channels to reach them. Keep your goals and resources in mind as you develop your plan. Key channels may include SEO (search engine optimization), PPC (pay-per-click ads), content marketing (blogs, articles, webinars), social media marketing, email marketing, text messaging, and various combinations.

In today's uber-competitive landscape, choosing the right channels for your goals and implementing an effective strategy can help to drive growth for your practice or medspa. The landscape is constantly evolving with new opportunities that can help drive more patients, especially the patients you want for your business, on the latest trends, tools, and best strategies will require a reasonable budget. You can start small with one or two keep programs, measure results and go from there. New opportunities and trends pop up all the time, so revisit your strategy frequently to make sure it is still effective and competitive.

DIGITAL DOMINATION

1. ***Target the right audience:*** *Digital marketing facilitates targeting specific demographics by their interests and behaviors, so your marketing efforts reach the most relevant audience.*
2. ***Market effectively:*** *Compared to print and consumer PR, you can allocate resources more efficiently to achieve higher ROI and easily make updates and changes.*
3. ***Build brand awareness:*** *A good digital marketing strategy can significantly increase brand awareness and credibility and helps companies establish a strong online presence.*
4. ***Expand your reach:*** *Reach a wider audience more efficiently to expand your client base from local to regional to global, and to tap into new markets.*
5. ***Measure success:*** *Through powerful analytics and data tracking, you can measure success for all your marketing strategies to make data-driven decisions.*

Traditional methods of acquiring new patients may not work as well or at all in some markets, so some practices have been forced to pivot to stay relevant and visible. Some patients are cautious in their choices and more concerned about outcomes and safety. Meanwhile, others may jump in without hesitation and are all about new, new, new. Then there are some who may take longer from their initial consultation to pull the trigger and commit to having a treatment.

First-time aesthetic patients may need multiple touchpoints, some reassurance, and a high comfort level before they sign on to have a treatment, especially if they are new to aesthetics. This may also be true among an older population of patients who may be newbies dipping a toe into aesthetic treatments. Offering a more personalized approach can be a sweet spot for attracting these patients and making them feel comfortable.

Having open and real conversations can help to build long-lasting trust and customer loyalty. This starts with listening to what patients are posting, commenting, and asking for. Building relationships directly with new patients based on a softer and less aggressive sales approach may serve you best.

The Trust Factor

Trust is the foundation of all relationships.

Of course, it is also important to be highly skilled, well-trained, experienced, knowledgeable, and trustworthy. In today's digital marketplace, patients also look for practitioners whom they can relate to and feel comfortable with. Adjectives like reliable, relatable, safe, caring, honest, experienced, and dedicated are words that are commonly found on rating sites.

No one wants to do business with someone they don't like or trust, especially when there are so many other practices to choose from in every market. Aesthetic patients can be bombarded with advice from friends and referrals who recommend "*using my doctor*" to curry favor with the practice they frequent.

The first place a prospective client may encounter your practice may be online through your website or social media platforms. These important touchpoints demonstrate who you really are as a professional by sharing genuine insights on your training specialty, team, clinic, and the entire client experience.

One of my personal pet peeves is the all too common overuse of tired stock photos that we see way too often. Replace them with real images and videos of the clinic team in action, with patients, doing treatments, etc. Add a personal touch and introduce yourself to prospective patients by sharing something about who you are as a medical professional and also as a person, parent, neighbor, etc.

Undoubtedly, digital marketing offers the most direct and effective method for lead generation at a lower cost and with measurable outcomes. Setting goals to diversify your marketing strategies and adopting more digital opportunities is the best way to future-proof your business.

(There has been a general shift in formats for content including for example, less text and more visuals like video, more targeted key messages, and a lighter, more entertaining tone.)

Ten Key Digital Marketing Tactics to Tap Into

1. **Content marketing is king**: Creating compelling videos, blogs, photos, images, and social posts to stimulate interest in products or services is critical to attracting users and keeping them coming back.
2. **Email marketing**: Email-based campaigns shared with a targeted list of recipients at select intervals are useful for maintaining awareness of what your practice offers and staying connected with patients.
3. **Focus on your audience**: Understand your target audience's wants and needs by creating content and campaigns that will resonate with them and produce the results you want to achieve.
4. **Measure and track ROI**: Monitor campaigns to measure the return on investment so you can allocate resources effectively. Track and analyze performance using tools like Google Analytics and social media site analytics. Adjust campaigns as needed for maximum results.
5. **Mobile marketing**: Advertising to promote products and services via mobile devices (phones and tablets).
6. **Pay-Per-Click (PPC)**: Invest in an ad strategy on key search engines (Google or Bing) to generate more clicks on your website and content.
7. **Personalization**: Personalize your marketing tactics based on your audience's preferences, behavior, and past interactions to enhance engagement and increase conversions.
8. **Search engine optimization**: SEO is still vital to increase your website visibility when users are searching for products or services on search engines (Google, Bing) to capture leads.
9. **Social media**: Utilize the most relevant apps your audience is active on as effective tools to reach potential clients and patients. Enhance your reach through an effective ad strategy, including boosting posts.
10. **Test and optimize**: Test the various aspects of your campaigns, including ads, artwork, messaging, subject lines, landing pages, and contests to identify what works best and optimize.

Putting Your Marketing Plan into Action

Building a marketing plan is a fundamental step towards maintaining and growing the connection between your brand and patients. This will also ensure that your strategies don't miss the mark.

Focus on what you do through a set of new channels, or existing channels that are constantly in a state of flux and being used in new ways.

Starting from a shared vision for your practice's brand can help to reflect what makes your brand stand out and be memorable.

This may require a new way of thinking. Understanding the current needs and desires of consumers requires carefully listening to the messages they are sharing. This also keep the practice team tapped into the products and treatments they are looking for to deliver high-level service.

Establishing a detailed understanding of your core customers positions your practice more accurately and allows the whole staff to address their evolving needs. Consumer behavior expectations can change practically overnight and accelerate the pace need to stay informed about important digital advancements. Understanding and acting on your clients' expectations will serve your well.

Leveraging Your Best Content

If you have good content to share, you can reformat some of it to nurture conversations through other platforms, such as blog posts, Instagram Live, webinars, Facebook communities, YouTube videos, stories, and more.

Listening closely to your patients' responses can provide vital clues as to their wants and needs. Keeping content useful and relevant to your target audience will help to maintain them. Format your content in the most appealing ways, for example, less text and more visuals, more targeted key messages, and a lighter, friendlier tone.

This suggests that you may not want to rely solely on the SEO or Google ads strategy that worked well for you last year to keep your treatment rooms busy. Voice search using the phones has become more popular for patients when searching for your clinic locally, as is social media.

Five Strategies for Success

1. Promote your practice and campaigns through a robust ad strategy.
2. Keep your website updated, with a monthly blog, SEO, and PPC (pay per click) campaigns.
3. Deploy monthly e-blasts with the right messages to target specific patient segments.
4. Monitor the days and times that your social channels get the most traffic to save your best content and boost the posts to get more eyes on them.
5. Invest more time and money in the top 2 or 3 platforms that are most popular among your target audience.

For example:

- Bring on a social media pro to manage it as a full-time job (not just a few hours per week)
- Take advantage of 'Meta Ads' for Instagram, Facebook as needed (WhatsApp and Messenger ads are also available)
- Follow smart tips and opportunities from 'TikTok for Business'
- Create and post short form and long form video content
- Engage with local influencers who are relatable to your patient audience

Driving Organic Traffic

As most of us have learned the hard way, Google is very fickle.

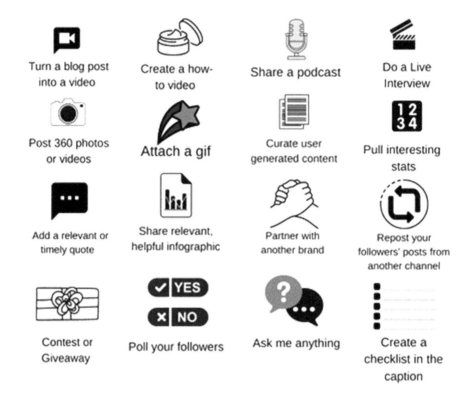

16 IDEAS FOR REPURPOSING CONTENT

Keeping your site updated with relevant and new information helps to get some love from search engines. Google tends to reward sites that regularly update content to gain more visitors or sites with higher rankings in search results. One way to stay in Google's good graces is to create consistently high-quality content.

SEO is data-dependent, and therefore the more metrics and data you track and analyze, the greater your chances of success. There are numerous SEO tools that can help with keyword research, competitive analysis, and content creation. For example, investing in affordable backlink tracking tools can help increase visibility.

Using long-tail keywords can also be a good strategy to help increase your content's visibility. These are specific phrases that people are more likely to use when searching for the products or services you offer.

Identify your practice's long-tail keywords and use them in titles, procedure descriptions, or blog post teasers to help boost your ranking in organic Google searches. For example, identify search terms with relatively low search volume and competition levels that may drive traffic to your site. As a rule, long-tail terms tend to be longer in length (three or more words) than other keyword types.

A prospective patient who has a specific concern may be more likely to search by incorporating that language:

- *"How to tighten my jowls" vs. "RF microneedling treatment"*
- *"I want to smooth my facial wrinkles" vs. just the words "filler" or "facelift"*

These keywords may also be beneficial for paid advertising campaigns since there may be less competition for more specific phrases which, in turn, influences pricing.

Boosting Content Through Optimization

To boost organic traffic, SEO and quality content are critical success strategies. On-page optimization may include using targeted keywords sparingly and naturally, without forcing them into content. It is also helpful to create appealing, eye-catching titles and to optimize your URLs to include your target keywords.

While you want to include keywords in your URLs, keep the URL as concise as possible. You can also include keywords in introductions, such as teasers or first lines of copy, rather than trying to fit them into every title which may make the content barely readable.

Content creation and SEO are time-consuming processes. Be prepared to take the amount of time required to achieve meaningful results. It can take several months or longer to rank your website organically, as you will be competing against other websites that may have been online for much longer.

As your SEO improves, it will hopefully continue to push your site higher and higher in the rankings over time. Supplementing your SEO efforts with paid search can speed up this process by covering both bases.

Building your presence on search engines requires a long-term commitment regarding resources, manpower, time, and money. Marketing strategies are not a perfect science and there is no guarantee that any of these methods with work for everyone every time. So, if you are not getting the results you were hoping for fast enough, either invest more time and money into your strategy, or rethink it.

These strategies should be an ongoing process. Don't just start a campaign and drop it when you don't get results as quickly as you anticipated. Even the best strategies require nurturing, patience, and a sufficient budget to move the needle.

Marketing is not a perfect science. It takes some trial and error to get you where you want to be. The only thing I will guarantee is that if you do nothing, you will find yourself in the same predicament next year and even five years from now.

Hyper-Personalized Communication

The more personalized and customized the content you leverage is, the more effective it will be to elevate your profile and keep your practice top of mind. Hyper-personalized communication vehicles can help to attract new customers and promote what your practice or medspa offers.

This may include everything from website copy, blogs, videos, photos, social media posts, e-books, messaging, ads, and any other strategy you may have tried to increase your online presence and attract more patients.

Unique content is the only way to go in this uber-competitive market. Google will punish you for duplicated content.

Personalizing your content to stay on brand and unique to your practice philosophy and image will raise your standing in your community. Continually analyze the copy you are putting out in all forms to make sure you are not deviating from the core messages you want patients to receive.

Caveat: While you may think getting content from a freelancer halfway across the world is a way to stretch your marketing budget, it may be costing you money in lost growth, and *missed opportunities to attract the right patients and build brand awareness.*

Best Practices for Using Text Messaging

Texting is a must to enhance customer service and connect with patients in a timely manner. If you are catering to Gen X, Y, and Z patients, it is pretty much essential.

Texting can be used for appointment scheduling, cancelations, rescheduling, prescriptions, skincare purchases, and general questions about treatments and aftercare. It can also be a huge time saver.

Choose a vendor that offers secure technology and two-way texting. Adhere to Health Insurance Portability & Accountability Act (HIPAA) in the US or General Data Protection Regulation (GDPR) in the EU, or the equivalent guidelines that govern your market.

Look for a system that can be used by physicians and medical staff to connect with patients without sharing their personal cell phone number.

Make sure patients understand the privacy risks that may arise from text messaging. The security of texts, even when encrypted, is not fool-proof and there is always a possibility of hacking. Request that patients text you back to acknowledge receipt of your message.

Adhere to the guidelines for patient privacy regulations that cover your market. For example, the HIPAA in the USA and the GDPR in the EU, or the equivalent organizations that apply in your market. To be safe, it may be wise to have patients sign a consent form digitally to opt into allowing your practice to connect through texting. Their consent should be kept on file and can be revoked at the patient's will at any time. It should include acknowledgment of the potential privacy risks and possible disclosure of information to third parties. Make sure no one in the practice uses any of the patient's identifying information (name, date of birth, address, etc.).

Caveat: *When texting patients, beware of the possibility of auto-corrections that can alter your message and potentially cause confusion with patients.*

Take Your Content Strategy to the Next Level

The more personalized the content you put out there is, the more effective it can be to elevate your profile and resonate with your target audiences. Hyper-personalized communications are key to attracting new customers and promoting what your practice offers. Content includes everything from website copy, blogs, videos, photographs, social media posts, e-books, brochures (if you are still using paper), messaging, ads, and anything else you are doing to increase your online presence to attract more patients.

There is no such thing as one-size-fits-all content creation. Unique content is the only way to go in today's competitive market. Personalizing your content to keep it on brand and unique to your practice philosophy and image will go a long way toward raising your standing in your community. Analyze the copy you are putting out there in all forms to determine whether it is on brand or deviating from the messages you want patients to get. If it is outdated or doesn't hit the right tone, you may need a content overhaul and brand refresh to stay up with the trends.

Enlist a team who understands the need for interesting, educational, and targeted content creation. Invest extra time and a decent budget to create a tailored experience that attracts more patients and the right patients to expand your practice.

Make sure that your content creator or freelancer is not creating content for your practice and many others. The Google gods won't take kindly to duplicate content and may punish you.

Mastering Email Marketing

Printed materials, brochures, forms, and postcards are so 2000.

Print has largely been replaced with email and text messaging that can get your message in front of your target audience in a matter of seconds and save you a lot of time and marketing funds. Stick with strategies designed to build relationships directly with patients that are based on their wants and needs.

You can never go wrong by taking a more personalized approach with patients who already know you. Sending the right message to the right people at the right time is a tried and true marketing tactic that is still in play right now.

Managing and curating your database is essential for success. For example, regularly check emails with patients as they arrive at your practice or medspa to stay current.

To be effective with email marketing, determine what you are trying to achieve. For example, what do you want the reader to do after they read your email? Make that your premium goal and stay on track.

Keeping your email marketing plan to a reasonable cadence, such as monthly, will help to prevent patients from opting out. The more personal you can make the content of your e-blasts, the better the chances are of getting recipients to actually read your messages and even share them with a friend to grow your database.

GET CAN-SPAM COMPLIANT

When drafting an email marketing campaign, you will need to investigate the rules and regulations established by the governing body in your market. For example, in the US, that would be the Federal Trade Commission (FTC), and in the UK, it is the Office of Fair Trading (OFT). Each campaign you create should be vetted to comply with these guidelines. Failure to do so may result in steep fines or other legal problems that can cost you big money and take time away from expanding your practice. Each email campaign you send should adhere to the compliance requirements that regulate your local market. Check with your local regulations to learn what laws apply to your patient outreach via emails and texting.

Six Ways to Stop Being an Unwitting Spammer

1. Use true header information.
2. All subject lines should be easily understood to avoid confusion.
3. Identify messages and content that are ads.
4. Include your location as needed.
5. Include clear opt-out information on every e-blast or text you send.
6. Handle opt-out requests automatically.

If you're not tracking results, you're not marketing effectively! It's too important to your bottom line to just guess...

Tracking and Evaluating

You need to know what is really working year after year so you can devote more time and energy to those tactics and weed out the ones that fall short. Tracking is essential to monitor the effectiveness of every marketing activity and to evaluate your overall plan. This is why digital tactics will add substantial value.

It is more efficient to track results from web traffic, Google ads, Facebook ads, and e-blasts than from print ads, media mentions, and billboards, for example. Any tactic that requires manual tracking may involve additional staff time, and measurements may be flawed.

You may include a dedicated phone line or code in a print ad to track the number of responses that come in, which may be handled by your marketing team or an external vendor who may need to calculate it manually. In a busy aesthetics practice, managing and caring for patients should always take top priority, which may necessitate farming out some of these chores.

We have worked with many practices that have had unsuccessful experiences outsourcing their marketing. In some cases, they chose the wrong vendors who did not understand their goals or had no experience in aesthetics or medical marketing.

If you don't find the right team, you may end up spending a lot more for an agency to learn how to market aesthetics on your tab. Before you enlist an external agency, check references, and make sure they have direct experience in medical aesthetics. You don't want to hire someone who needs to learn the ropes on your time.

There is no substitute for direct experience in your field. Just because a marketing group has done websites or a social strategy for a construction company or a clothing store, does not mean that they are qualified to understand the nuances of medical aesthetics practices.

WHEN SHOULD YOU OUTSOURCE SOME OF YOUR MARKETING?

If you don't have enough staff – or the right staff – to dedicate the requisite time needed to design a cohesive marketing plan and stick with it, you basically have three options:

1. *Hire an experienced full-time or part-time marketing manager for your practice or medspa.*
2. *Enlist the services of an external specialist or agency that can guide you through the process of creating a marketing plan to address your specific needs and goals and can carry on executing it for you.*
3. *The hybrid option is to enlist an external agency that reports to your internal team.*

Ideally, my recommendation is to have a dedicated staff member (or members) aided by an experienced external agency to help design and execute your marketing plan for best results. This strategy affords you the best of both worlds.

Think Global, Act Local

It is unrealistic to think that you can attract everyone, and why would you want to?

Segmenting your target audience will serve to guide you on where to devote your resources and what promotional methods and key messages to run with.

Plan to target your most likely patients through the process of market segmentation. Segment the audience you most want to reach so you can better target them with what you have to offer.

Identify and reach out to the target audience(s) to find new groups of potential patients. For example, men, millennials, people of different skin types, hair restoration candidates, intimate health candidates, etc.

You may also segment patients by demographics (age, gender, ethnicity, marital status) and/or by psychographics (lifestyle, values, needs, wants).

Working as a team, create action steps that detail how the marketing variables of product, price, place, and promotion can be used to develop a marketing plan through key objectives and overall strategies.

Your marketing mix should serve as the basis for your plan. Define every treatment, product, and service you offer in terms of what it is, what it does, who the target audience is, advantages, benefits, solutions, and alternatives. Set pricing for each line item on your plan based on a competitive analysis.

Consider how you want to promote the most lucrative and popular treatments, products, and services you offer. Most practices do not have an unlimited budget to aggressively promote everything they offer, and You shouldn't do that even if you can.

Prioritize the treatments that you want to do more. For example, you may be able to generate more revenue from big-ticket laser treatments and injectables vs. facials and skincare treatments. Aim to attract more patients who can afford to go for a series of RF microneedling rather than just any old microneedling pen.

Develop Partnerships within Your Community

Teaming up with like-minded local businesses is always a good idea. Seek out potential opportunities to partner with complementary shops and vendors to promote your clinic. This is a way to share your resources with a non-competitive business for cross-promotion.

For example, select a partner with a complementary business (not a direct competitor) in your area that has a similar customer base to your own to create a collaborative special offer. This could be a cool gym or yoga studio, a popular hair and makeup salon, a luxe clothing shop, a wine shop, etc. Each business should leverage their own database to promote this special offer and event.

Another option is to team up with other professionals with whom you may share clients. For instance, an aesthetic clinic may partner with a cosmetic dentist or plastic surgeon. This strategy can help build up both businesses and foster relationships that may lead to more referrals and collaborations in the future.

People tend to appreciate taking part in something that benefits their local community. Try hosting a give-back event during your slow season. Donate a portion of sales for a specific day or selected service or product to your favorite local charity.

This feel-good strategy can help to raise your profile within your community and spread goodwill. You can expect more referrals to follow too.

DIGITAL ADVERTISING TIPS FROM THE WEBTOOLS GROUP

- *Many patients end up searching Google, mostly on their phones, when they start looking for a provider for the cosmetic condition they would like to address. The cost per click or per lead tends to be very high, which means the budget needs to be managed professionally, and ineffective campaigns should be shut off.*
- *Google tends to be very restrictive. For example, it will not allow a website that mentions 'platelet rich plasma (PRP)' to advertise as they consider it an "experimental" treatment. Google will often ask you to show them a letter of permission before you can run ads that contain the word "BOTOX," because it is a drug.*
- *As Google can decide it will not show your ads to the whole audience, in many cases it results in ineffective campaigns. Your ad manager needs to know how to check and make sure the ads are not restricted, and how to work with their Google rep on addressing limitations.*
- *It is important to diversify your online lead sources. YouTube works well with short, visually engaging videos, especially for surgical procedures. If the ad is approved (ads on each of these platforms are required to go through an approval process), it may result in leads at a lower cost than Google. To measure ROI, capture all leads and calculate the total revenue generated by the leads who converted to treatments, divided by the cost of the ads and management fees.*
- *On Instagram, stay updated with recent Meta restrictions on using before-and-after photos if approved. Short videos in your feed can be boosted. You can test different posts and based on the results choose the ones to fund. Patients may message you on Instagram, so it is important that someone responds and communicates by direct message on Instagram with potential patients before they switch to a phone call.*
- *Facebook is still popular in many countries. It is sometimes preferred by more mature consumers, **who** can be a great source of patients interested in age-reversing treatments. Ads are based on recorded Facebook Live segment. Ads can be connected to a form which potential patients can fill out right after seeing the ad, without leaving the Facebook app.*
- *TikTok's ad platform allows you to choose who to target, and the cost per "serious" lead tends to be lower than Google in some markets. Try to create short, attention-grabbing video content that can be "boosted" as an ad.*

- *Resources are always limited, so it is better to add one marketing channel at a time, whether it is Google ads, SEO, or email marketing. Partner with a consultant or an agency that specializes in the beauty and aesthetics vertical and put a six-month plan together. It often takes a few months to work out the kinks and see a good return on investment.*
- *Diversify your sources of new patients so you are less dependent on any one channel. The digital landscape is changing rapidly, and it is best to experiment with new platforms when they start gaining popularity – this is the time you can leap to stardom.*
- *SEO for medical and aesthetic clinics is more complex than ever. Google looks at experience, expertise, authoritativeness, and trustworthiness when it decides how to rank your website in search results. These signals are derived from your items like your online reputation and medical publications. Work with an SEO professional to adhere to Google's ever-evolving guidelines.*

Source: https://webtoolsgroup.com/

4

Optimizing the Marketing Mothership

You realize our mistrust of the future makes it hard to give up the past.

Chuck Palahniuk, author of *Survivor*

Three seconds.

That's how much time most new visitors will spend on your website. So, if you don't catch their attention in those three seconds, they may be lost forever.

A professional-looking and functioning website design is a critical success factor for building your online presence, but that is just the beginning. You also need well-organized, dynamic content that will attract and engage visitors so they will spend more time on your site.

The copy should be designed to convert visitors to learn enough about you and what you offer to ultimately become customers. This goal requires giving visitors a memorable experience on your site. Develop your site to be consistent with your practice location, facility, and be on brand. It also needs to stand out from all the competition.

Every component of your site serves as a reflection of you, your business, and your brand. It will determine what prospective patients think about you, and how they feel about you. Well-crafted copy has the power to start a conversation with visitors that will lead to a consultation, whether virtual or live in your practice.

Before you start writing your copy or assigning someone to write it for you, understand what your visitors want and need. This will help you keep the conversation all about them instead of just about you.

Great unique content can help win the hearts, minds, and wallets of the patients you are most interested in attracting.

Websites to Help You Ace Your Bottom Line

Despite the rise of social media channels for creating brand awareness, a robust modern website is still an essential component of an effective marketing strategy.

This is especially true if you want to attract patients and clients of all ages and stages.

You may never know what the weapon of choice may be for each patient you want to attract, so it is wise to cover all your bases.

Eight Components of a Killer Website

1. Your site should be set up to be mobile-friendly, as most people search on their phones or tablets vs. on their laptops.
2. Ensure that your site loads quickly to avoid users opting out.
3. Simplify your site's navigation and search to make it easy for visitors to find what they are looking for quickly and effectively.

DOI: 10.1201/9780429356742-4

4. Optimize your content to grab more attention from search engines.

5. Eye-catching visuals help to keep viewers engaged. Invest in photos from a photoshoot or, if possible, photos of some of your most photogenic patients instead of stock photos. Build up a robust portfolio of before-and-after photos with patient permission in writing to keep on file.

6. Curate videos of patients talking about their experience to demonstrate the benefits of a series or ongoing program in your practice or medspa. This can be a good workaround in markets where patient photos are not permitted.

7. If possible, display results at specific intervals; number of days and weeks to educate patients on the healing process, aftercare, and the final results they can expect.

8. Real patients are more relatable to your local audience because their praise is authentic and more trusted than paid influencers. Include comments, videos, testimonials, thank you notes, and praise from real patients on your site.

Hyper-Personalized Communication

The more personalized and custom content you put out there, the more effective it will be at elevating your profile and keeping your practice top of mind. Hyper-personalized communications vehicles can help to attract new customers and promote what your practice or medspa offers.

This may include everything from website copy, blogs, videos, photos, social media posts, e-books, messaging, ads, and anything else you may be using to increase your online presence and attract more patients.

Unique content is the only way to stand out in today's competitive market.

Personalizing your content to stay on brand and unique to your practice philosophy and image will raise your standing in your community. Analyze the copy that you are putting out in all forms to make sure it is not deviating from the messages you want patients to get.

Why You Need a Chatbot

By now, unless you are living under a rock, you will have heard about OpenAI, the original project that brought AI into our lives, founded by Elon Musk (of Tesla and X) and Sam Altman (the tall nerdy guy who warned the US Congress of the potential dangers of AI).

ChatGPT hails from OpenAI. It was designed to generate "human-like" responses to questions or information. Thus, it is being used for conversational applications, such as virtual assistants and chatbots.

If you have ever shopped online or booked a flight or hotel, you have been exposed to chatbots. They are now routinely used for all forms of customer service functions. These are now readily deployed as instant messengers on websites to answer questions and FAQs online. They are getting more prevalent and smarter all the time.

For more in-depth info on this, refer to Chapter 9.

The Benefits of Adopting a Chatbot

Chatbots have emerged as an essential component of a modern and functional website. The technology is constantly improving to be more sophisticated and personalized, giving each client a different experience. For example, they can be programmed for your specific needs such as asking customers what they need help with and sharing a list of options for clients to choose from.

There is really no limit to what a chatbot can do, and the benefits far exceed the costs involved in setting them up. Programming an intelligent chatbot is like having your office open 24/7 for patients to get answers to simple, more specific queries.

Clients are now acclimated to dealing with chatbots in a wide range of everyday businesses such as airlines, hotels, banks, and many other service industries. Customizing what your bot can say and do helps to keep up with patient needs and demands.

You may start with basic tasks, such as, "Where is the office located?" or "Is there parking nearby?" and go from there.

Your chatbot can be programmed to take on many more complex tasks, such as:

- *Do you take insurance and which ones?*
- *Do you offer a specific treatment?*
- *What skincare brands do you have?*
- *When is the next appointment available?*
- *Can I get laser hair removal in your clinic?*
- *I want to reschedule, cancel, or book an appointment.*
- *What days are Nurse Suzi working?*

By now, consumers have become accustomed to engaging with bots, and their capabilities are skyrocketing. For example, chatbots can help to resolve common service issues like refunds or appointment cancellations. In some cases, they can be programmed to customize recommendations for products and even schedule appointments.

Conversational AI is taking it to the next level. For example, you can get an answer to many queries in a quick minute rather than staying on hold for minutes to hours awaiting the opportunity to speak with a real human – I mean the flesh and blood kind.

The myriad of benefits include reducing the workload of office personnel, responding in real-time to patient queries, directing more complex questions to medical personnel when needed, and being available to take calls and direct patients to the right person within the practice.

There is really no limit to what a chatbot can do anymore. The benefits far exceed the costs involved in setting up a system for your business.

This is true for all patient segments today. Even more mature or less tech-savvy patients understand how to deal with a chatbot, and those who are timid about it will have to learn post haste.

Over time, the technology has become more accessible, affordable, and customizable. Your practice's chatbot can be quite different from that of your competitors' chatbot if that is your goal is to stand out.

8 THINGS YOU NEED TO KNOW ABOUT CHATBOTS

- Chatbot technology – also referred to as Virtual Assistants – are found everywhere from your personal to your business life.
- They are the precursors to artificial intelligence (AI).
- Not all chatbots are equipped with AI yet, but many or most of them are in the process of converting.
- Chatbots are used for all forms of customer service from airlines to medspas – Add a 'Go Live' or 'Speak to a representative' button.
- They can use conversational AI (like ChatGPT) to better understand users' queries and answer more relevant queries.
- They are readily used as 'instant messengers' on websites to answer FAQs.
- Check out your favorite news sites and retailers for more ideas on how to use AI driven chatbots for your practice.
- Smart speakers at home like SMS platforms, Amazon's Alexa, Facebook's WhatsApp and Messenger, and other models we use for work and personal communication use chatbots in one form or another.

Unique Content Strategy

The more personalized the content that you put out there is, the more effective it can be to elevate your profile and resonate with your target audiences. Hyper-personalized communications are key to attracting new customers and promoting what your practice offers. Content includes everything from website copy, blogs, videos, photographs, social media posts, e-books, brochures (if you are still using paper), messaging, ads, and anything else you are doing to increase your online presence to attract more patients.

Chose a vendor with experience working with medical professionals and who understands the pervasive need unique, and educational, content creation. Invest in extra time and a decent budget to get exceptional copy, graphics and content creation that attracts more patients and the kind of patients you want to have in your practice.

You may think the strategy of using content created by a freelancer halfway across the world is saving you money, but in fact, it may be doing the reverse. It can cost you money in lost growth, new patients, more treatments, decimating your brand, and many more opportunities.

Content creator or freelancer is not creating duplicate content for your practice as well as many others.

Be sure that your content creator or freelancer is not creating duplicate content for your practice as well as many others, which is a common dilemma. Is the person charged with creating your content for blogs, social media, your website, and consumer-facing materials, working for loads of your competitors too? Find out because Google doesn't like duplicate content and may punish you for it, plus you don't want to see your content on someone else's site. This is violation. Random freelancers may not to be up to speed on the rules governing physicians or medspas and the nuances of the doctor-patient relationship.

Setting Clear Goals

To ensure that you choose the best tactics to meet your marketing goals, get clear about what those goals are.

Consider both your short-term and long-term goals:

- *What are your key priorities and timeline?*
- *Are you trying to expand your online presence, generate more leads, attract more patients interested in having treatments or surgery, or all of the above?*
- *Are you on a mission to build up your practice for more repetitive non-surgical treatments, injectables, exosomes, microneedling, and/or other energy-based devices?*
- *Are you keen to drive more interest in spa services?*
- *Is attracting a new market sector, such as male patients or Gen Z, top of mind?*
- *What does success look like for your personal business goals?*

This will help you define all the components that belong in your marketing plan for delivery in the next quarter or year. Schedule regular brainstorming sessions with the whole clinic staff and marketing team to review key messages and timelines, and keep everyone who has a say in the loop.

Evaluate how you are planning marketing tactics, including monthly specials, offers, events, webinars, blog posts, and social media content. Plan your key messages based on the services you offer, and then decide how to differentiate them from your competition.

For example, perhaps you want to add a new energy-based system, filler, or skincare brand in the next quarter. Start planning early by designating the steps leading up to launching the treatment and marketing to your existing patients first.

Checklist for Adding a New Treatment

- Start early (four to six weeks out) drafts of a comprehensive plan to make it official.
- Share your plan and assign tasks to all stakeholders in the practice or medspa so everyone takes part in the launch.
- Determine pricing for single sessions vs. packages.
- Generate excitement with patients about "what's coming next" – aesthetic patients love to learn about something new and "be the first" to try it.
- Add information about the new treatment to the landing page of your website. Ask the vendor to share images you can use before you have any of your own.
- Spread the word on your website, blog, e-blasts, social channels, signage in your facility, videos, etc.
- Whenever possible, allow staff to experience, or at least watch, the new treatment or product being introduced so they can speak to patients with knowledge and credibility.
- Create a limited one-time offer where the first (X amount – 10 or 20 as you wish) of clients who sign up will get (20% and up) to capture an early revenue stream and gain experience with the treatment.
- Keep the momentum going through a robust integrated marketing plan. Collect patient photos to share if possible and maintain excitement about the new treatment by showcasing what it offers and the results

The Aesthetics Marketing Funnel

In its simplest form, there is a funnel that happens to someone buying your product or service.

At the very top of the funnel, they might not have any need for your product or service yet or at all. However, you still want to make an impression on every prospective client for the time when their status changes and they are ready to commit to having a treatment or buying a product in your practice.

The theory is that when they do need you, they will remember you. However, that will only happen if your marketing, positioning, and what you offer are memorable and your messaging resonates and strikes the right emotions.

The overall goal is to consistently influence as many potential clients as possible. The more you do, the more likely it is that some will remember you over all the other clinics and practices in the market.

Figures 4.1 and 4.2 show the stages and tactics for an Aesthetics Marketing Funnel.

Traffic Does Not Always Bring More Conversions

More traffic doesn't necessarily translate into more sales or conversions. In other words, not all traffic is created equal.

It is understandable to think that because you are getting more traffic, you will have more sales. There can be some correlations, but there is no guarantee. The difference is targeted traffic.

You can have a thousand hits a day from random visitors, but if they are not interested in what you offer, that traffic will not help you fill your treatment rooms. However, when you get traffic from targeted clients, the difference can be huge.

This can get lost sometimes when focusing only on website traffic and not on the quality and intent of visitors.

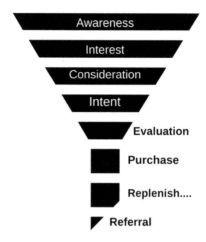

FIGURE 4.1   Aesthetics marketing funnel - 8 stages

-AWARENESS
Marketing campaigns, Google, friends, media
-**INTEREST**
Events, ads, webinars, social media, search, video
-**CONSIDERATION**
Engage with emails, targeted content, text messaging
-**INTENT** Product info, specials, case studies
-**EVALUATION** Demos/videos, samples, sales aids
-**PURCHASE** Marketing and sales to prove the
value/benefits of your products & services
-**REPLENISH** Post sale of products/treatments, drive
follow up through consistent engagement across
channels
-**REFERRAL** Incentive clients/patients to become
advocates and send their friends/family

FIGURE 4.2   Aesthetic marketing funnel - tactics

TECHNOLOGY IS YOUR BFF

There is a plethora of new tools, channels, and technological advances that turn up in our inboxes daily. The fast pace of digital marketing and communication presents challenges for busy doctors, managers, and consultants to keep up with all the trends. However, it is important to stay on top of the trends and be ready to adapt swiftly when innovations that have the potential to revolutionize the way we communicate and work pop up.

For those of us who are not "techies" by nature (that includes me!), new technologies, systems, and automation may present challenges beyond our capabilities. The more you can automate systems in your business, the more efficient you can be, which ultimately makes for a happier staff as well as a better bottom line.

Don't despair!

For every new development, you can find the right experts to help you with whatever you need to keep your business running smoothly. But don't wait till another disaster happens. Have these pros in place NOW, if only for peace of mind.

My go-to supports include the team from Apple for Small Business (I think they know us by first names by now), and the global team at Webtools, who are always at the ready to help us.

MOBILE MARKETING TIPS FROM WEBTOOLS DIGITAL MARKETING GROUP

- *Once per quarter, give some TLC to your treatment pages. Add new videos of you or patients talking about their experience, refresh the before-and-after photos featured on the page, and update the text. Both Google and patients will see you as an expert in that treatment, and you are likely to receive more inquiries as a result.*
- *Automate your marketing by developing drip campaigns. Based on each patient's journey, you can automatically send them a series of emails and text messages to further educate them about the treatment they are interested in, such as a link to watch a webinar you recorded on the topic. Throughout the campaign, have call-to-action buttons for booking consultations or communicating with staff. You only need to design that campaign once, and it will constantly generate new patients from cold leads.*
- *Tools like Google Analytics can help you identify issues on your website. Does a high percentage of visitors leave after visiting a certain page? Was there a recent drop in visits from one of your traffic sources? Are there pages that better convert visitors to leads? Tweak your website as if it is gardening work – small improvements add up and results are always measurable.*
- *Experiment with new website features by running A/B tests. Only if you see that metrics improved with that new gizmo, should you incorporate it into all pages.*
- *When you redo your website, ask the designer to work on a mobile-first design. Since most people will see the website on a phone or a tablet, the focus should be on their experience. Users should be able to easily read texts and navigate through pages.*
- *Add customized call-to-action buttons for mobile phones. These are designed to make it highly visible and easy to call your office, send a text message, or book an appointment online.*
- *Design ad campaigns that will focus on mobile users – geolocating them on the go with ads that render well on phones. The ads can be linked to your reviews and ratings from GoogleMyBusiness. When potential patients click on the ads, they should visit a relevant mobile-friendly landing page.*
- *Encourage patients to share their experience on your GoogleMyBusiness listing, as it is highly visible on phones when patients search Google locally.*
- *Develop a list of patients' phone numbers with signed consent from each of them. Based on local regulations, you may be able to send them SMS campaigns to present new devices and treatments, offer timely promotions, and other messages designed to increase the number of annual visits to the practice*

Source: https://www.webtoolsgroup.com

5

Content Marketing Pearls for Platforms

Great ideas are a dime a dozen. It's executional skills that are rare.

Kevin O'Leary, Shark Tank

The overriding goal of content marketing is to get your content in front of the right audience at the right time.

Great, unique, and memorable content adds value to everything you do as a company or brand. It can help to attract patients and clients and to share solutions for their problems and concerns.

You can use content to make connections and build communities. For example, while social media, email marketing, and text messaging are important ways to connect with patients, creating communities can open new doors for your brand. The concept of community is at the forefront of digital marketing strategies as more people want to reach out, get support from other users, and weigh in on topics that matter to them. People want to feel like they are engaged with brands and individuals who share values in line with their own.

From editorial copy, website content, blog posts, and social media posts, everything you put out there for your brand should be consistent in tone and quality. The more unique and memorable your content is, the more engagement you can achieve. Create meaningful and unique content that adds value to your audience.

> *The most effective content is searchable, shareable, consumable, and most importantly relevant to your brand and TARGETED audience.*

As visitors become more interested in the value of your brand, your reach will expand. Ideally, a highly engaged audience may be encouraged to share some of your content with their own communities, which can help to expand your database over time.

Omnichannel Marketing

Omnichannel marketing is self-explanatory (Figure 5.1).

If you have a Facebook and Instagram business account, plus an optimized website with a robust blog, essentially you are practicing some form of omnichannel marketing.

While that does not mean your plan is sufficient to keep your treatment rooms full in the current competitive climate, it's just a good start.

Marketing technology can create, execute, manage, and measure the performance of content – both online and offline – campaigns, and experiences. It can be a very effective way to streamline the customer journey and implement an omnichannel marketing strategy.

If you are having a tough time keeping up with the constant stream of new developments in marketing tactics, you're not alone. A common complaint we hear from practices is that they get onto a cool platform and invest time, effort, and money only to find that a new and improved technology platform turned up a few months or years later just when you've finally got the hang of it.

News flash: There will always be a new and improved, hot technology popping up that will catch your eye but that doesn't mean that you have to start all over again.

DOI: 10.1201/9780429356742-5

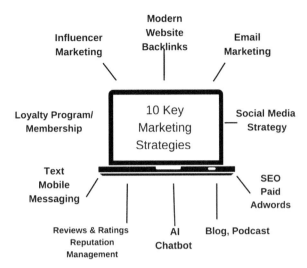

FIGURE 5.1 Omnichannel marketing.

Practitioners are keen to invest in the newest technology in the hopes that it will make their lives easier, faster and cheaper. They are often drawn to sophisticated tech that claims to help you gather and store data and use that data for marketing and decision-making.

Driving Real Connections

Creating unique and effective content is an integral part of an effective digital marketing and brand-building plan. This may include producing written, audio, or visual information for content marketing platforms, websites, social channels, blogs, and e-books.

The best content should strike the right balance to reach your target audiences with the right messages, ideal format, with the right tone and eye-catching visuals you need to communicate the precise messages you want to deliver in an informative way. When you post just any old content that doesn't feel personal or informative, it may have the reverse effect by undermining what you are trying to achieve. A common mistake is to post anything you have because you think you need to be active on every channel to be seen. Please resist the temptation! Weak or poor content may be more detrimental than posting no content at all.

The content you put out into the universe should have an end goal in mind, such as targeting a specific audience like affluent women over 40. It should stimulate a response, such as following your Instagram, visiting your website, making an appointment, purchasing a skincare product, or sharing the content with a friend.

For example, consider a newsletter in the form of an email to be delivered to your subscribers that provides important announcements. Newsletters are most actionable when your organization has an email service provider through which to send the newsletter and measure its impact, such as Mailchimp or ConstantContact. These platforms are essential to create and manage newsletter campaigns and announcements to your active clients, and track opens rates and opt-outs seamlessly.

THE BENEFITS OF E-BOOKS

Creating e-books on popular topics is a frequently overlooked strategy that we have had great success with. These are booklets, typically in a PDF format, that are hyper-focused on a timely topic of interest to your target audience. To download the e-book, the visitor must give something in consideration, for example, their email. In some cases, you may want to add more specifics to get for future marketing purposes, such as name, address, age (by group), and an indication of their interest in a list of procedures on offer in your practice. This can prove to be an effective and affordable way to expand your database.

Patient-Facing Marketing

There is a big difference in tone, imagery, and messaging when developing content for the purpose of promoting sales as in treatments or products, as opposed to creating content to engage, entertain, and develop deep connections with the audience.

Social media channels are by far the most valuable patient-facing marketing tools we can tap into. To empower your social team to succeed with relationship-building, they will need to select the most important social channels based on the target audience.

Designating a healthy mix of original content paired with curated content that your followers will be interested in seeing can work effectively. If the content resonates with the right audience in the right way, it can educate viewers on the core strengths of your brand. This, in turn, can help to attract more visitors, shares, and user engagement.

The next step would be to drive conversations that encourage users to share your content with their fans and followers.

Six Ideas for Creating Shareable Content

1. Third-party research and clinical studies.
2. Press releases or news announcements.
3. Video interviews and blogs.
4. Podcasts featuring staff members, special guests, colleagues, etc.
5. Relevant statistics from legitimate sources (medical societies, hospitals, news outlets, published studies).
6. Timely news items with a local or regional angle.

Everyone craves interesting, unique, and entertaining content. Curating compelling content in any form from legitimate sources and making sure to credit the original sources, can keep your audience engaged and elevate your platform.

The Value of Influencers

Influencers can also play a huge role in your marketing strategy. The trick is to find the right ones with loyal, devoted followers who take their advice on recommendations for products and service

In some cases, one great post from an influencer to follower can make or break your ROI. Try to form a relationship with the influencer in person before making any commitment.

Micro-influencers who are local to your market can be very effective even though they may have a much smaller following. If they are within a short distance from your practice or medspa, they will have a more relevant following of prospective new patients interested in what you offer.

Before working with any influencers, they need to be vetted to make sure they have the right following for the patients you want to attract and are aspirational and relatable to your target audience. In general, local influencers may be the most beneficial for your practice goals and affordable, rather than someone who is halfway across the world and may be irrelevant to your primary audience.

If your organic reach has fallen below a certain threshold, such as 25 to 50 thousand followers, you may need to pay to drive more exposure for your brand. In some cases, influencers with large followings may become digital marketing agencies themselves, and can make money from numerous endorsements and affiliate links from parnerships.

For example, if an Instagrammer writes about how much she loves the Hydrafacial® treatment she had in your clinic, some of her followers might click through to check it out online. This is where having an affiliate link can be a win-win for the practice and the influencers.

To achieve the best results, take time to develop a deep understanding of the influencer's target audience and then design campaigns that are most likely to resonate with that specific audience. Keep in mind that consumers are demanding transparency across all channels

PAY TO PLAY

Make sure that you are following the local regulations regarding working with influencers. They may ask for free treatments, cash, or both or nothing at all. Keep in mind that if you do any free treatments or pay influencers for their post, in most countries or regions, you will be expected to make sure they post the requisite words required, such as: #ad #advert #advertisement #sponsored, etc. In some markets, like the USA and UK, fines or reprimands may apply.

The Rise of Creators

The demand for unique, original, fresh, and likeable content has no limits. It's not just about having more content, but rather creating better content that adds value to your audience so they will be loyal and send their friends to engage with your content to grow your social channels. Content creators are an emerging and important category of professionals whose job is to produce written, audio, or video content to connect with a specific audience on an increasingly wide range of marketing platforms. These may include social channels, blogs, websites, and more.

The content they produce may be in the form of a testimonial on Instagram, a blog post for your practice website, a video for YouTube to promote skincare products, plus countless other uses. The opportunities are only limited to their creativity, your goals and your budget.

Creators "create" original content to target a specific, predetermined audience to generate an agreed upon response. This can also be a wide range of one or more goals. For example, to generate more followers on social channels, engage with existing followers to encourage sales, then reach out to their network to drive new followers to the client's site or channel. The possibilities are endless.

They will often create content to target a selected audience and evoke a response, such as new followers, more site visits, sales of products, or gift cards. Many creators are looking for 'brand partnerships' as opposed to 'sponsorships' that align with their voice, image, and followers, so their posts will look and feel natural rather than contrived like an ad.

Bottom Line: *Check out A Creator's Guide to Instagram by Instagram to get ideas:* https://www.instagram.com/creators/

Tips for Working with Creators

Working with creators is like enlisting an external team to help elevate your brand on specific social channels. Depending on the creator and how you contract with them, they can be a game changer for your social media chops.

Professional content creators, or "creators" as they are called, are like the new influencers. They are in demand for their unique talent, originality, and passion for effectively communicating messages to the right social media audiences at the right time. The advantage of working with creators is tapping into their 'creativity' and the deep connections within their networks.

As some of these creators may be young and new to the world of injectables and breast implants, make your goals and expectations crystal clear from the outset. Provide direction in terms of your brand, style, and positioning as well as the specific audiences you want to gain traction with. If the creator is reasonably local, invite them to your practice to learn what you do and meet the whole team. Explain the rules governing patient privacy at the outset.

There is a lot of content with varying degrees of accuracy and creativity on every channel. Be careful to work with influencers and content creators who get your mission and understand your brand. If you align your content with the wrong influencer, who does not have the right targeted audience, it can undermine your brand and waste your marketing funds.

Many creators want to grow and expand. They may seek out long-term brand partnerships (rather than just one-off sponsorships) that align with their content, so their posts feel natural. They often prefer working with brands and companies to offer guidance and support, rather than just leave them to it.

This strategy reinforces that you are a good listener, rather than just being interested in sharing your own opinions or posting images of your designer bags or decadent vacations. In fact, it can be better to come across as less self-serving by unveiling a different side of your personality.

Showing that you are interested in what others are doing and having dialogues with people with unique voices will add more depth to your feed. This demonstrates that you are part of a community, so it's not just all about you.

Taking Care of Business

It is important to set project goals from the very beginning. Just like working with influencers, a detailed contract should be drafted for both parties to sign before embarking on a project. The document should include an NDA (Non-Disclosure Agreement), scope of work, terms, deliverables, payment, timelines, and revisions. If the work product is intended to live on the creator's social channel or channels, those specifics should be included as well as an approximate date to go live and for how long. The contract should also include an exit clause if the relationship does not work out.

Using Creators to Elevate Your Brand

Assign someone on your marketing team to develop a relationship with the creator and to be responsible for managing the process. Share a brand book that carefully maps out the style and tone of the communications you want to achieve. This should include key messages, look, and feel. If they are creating content for placement on your channels, the style and imagery should be consistent for each piece of content they craft to stay on brand.

If it is your first time working with the creator, share some examples of what great content looks like to you, as well as what you want to avoid. Visuals will make these points much clearer than just words. Provide specific goals to evaluate the process without stifling their creative juices too much.

Make sure the creator has an open line of communication with a team member to answer questions as they arise. Creatives tend to have their own style and work process, so be prepared to let them do their thing at their own pace. However, put deadlines and guidelines in place. For example, creating a series of videos may take longer than just text-based material.

When working with well-known creators, leverage their popularity. Let your brand and mission fit into their style rather than the other way around. If you ask them to change their style to fit the brand, you may sour the relationship. Their followers may also lose interest in the content they are putting out, which would defeat its purpose.

Giving Feedback Gently

Sometimes getting the right messages across can be tricky in the healthcare and aesthetics categories, so ground rules should be established from the outset.

In some cases, the shared content they turn out may not hit the right tone early in the relationship. There are many reasons why their shared content may not hit the right tone early in the relationship. There may have been a misunderstanding over instructions that are too open to interpretation. Providing feedback gently will help guide their work without causing any ill will or undesired upsets. One or two rounds of feedback are reasonable. If more is needed, re-examine the path of communication to improve efficiency. When the relationship isn't working, it is prudent to just move on.

As with influencers, who may have tens to hundreds of thousands of followers, try not to break up with a creator with a high level of notoriety on a sour note. Many of them consider themselves to be "artists" and take their craft very seriously.

When the relationship is on good terms, it can lead to generating great content that truly delivers results for your practice.

New Rules for Content Marketing

Whether it's native advertising, sponsored editorial content, or blog posts, creating and sharing great content is the key to success in digital marketing.

Simply having a website and social media platforms is not enough anymore to stand out from the pack. Your marketing plan also requires some creative and engaging content that can promote your practice in fresh, new ways. Content marketing is all about getting your content in front of the right audience at the right time.

In theory, content marketing is designed to create valuable, relevant, and compelling information on a consistent basis for a targeted audience with the goal of stimulating activity and results for your company or brand. Ultimately, your content should aim to build an audience that likes, trusts, and respects your brand.

Custom content marketing is on the rise, mainly because Google has increased the viability of content. In short, custom content is real, brand-specific content demonstrating your expertise through a range of modalities, including infographics, videos, photos, articles, podcasts, and blog posts.

Marketing professionals need to ensure that all the generated content integrates seamlessly with their marketing activities and business goals. Content should never exist just for its own sake. It should be well thought out, address the needs of your clients, and effectively move them closer towards making a purchasing decision.

For example, keeping up a blog on your website is still a great way to produce custom content in-house on a regular basis.

Be a Good Storyteller

Think of yourself as the storyteller whose job is to inform and inspire your audience to drive measurable actions that impact your bottom line. From editorial copy, website content, blog posts, and social media posts, everything you put out there for your brand should be consistent in tone and quality. The best content is searchable, shareable, consumable, and relevant.

Your main objectives should include raising your brand's profile and messaging as well as promoting lead generation, decision-making, retention, and ultimately, driving purchasing decisions. Raising awareness can be effectively accomplished via content, social media, and video marketing. Lead generation is more typically linked to direct search and digital advertising.

More brands that formerly spent their budgets on traditional advertising are devoting a big chunk of their budgets to investing in relevant content to connect with their target audiences. Branded content is different than what is known as "native advertising." Native advertising is a type of format that directs users to branded content, whereas branded content is a fresh form of marketing that is more closely aligned with the objectives of traditional marketing strategies.

This trend is in part driven by the realization that most consumers don't like to be sold to. Consumers are programmed to do research online before making a purchasing decision or ever reaching out to your practice. If you are lacking in rich content to persuade them to reach out, they may bolt and find other sources that are waiting in the wings to engage them.

Your Own Online Experience

How do you digest content?

- *Are you turned off by a hard-sell approach?*
- *Are you more likely to respond when a product pitch is data-driven?*

Guess What?

Those traits just mean you are human. Well, so is your target audience.

Try not to bombard them with bluster, chest-pounding, overtly salesy content that adds no value to them and is likely to turn them off.

Instead of aggressively pitching your products and services, providing truly relevant and useful content to your target audience and offering them solutions for what is on their minds may be a better strategy. You don't always need to heavily incorporate brand messaging and product pitches to make an impact.

Branded content should be a mix of different types, including content designed to generate brand awareness, sponsored editorial content for specific promotions, and educational content to highlight a new technique or patient experience, and much more.

Knowing your target audience intimately helps to design a content experience that offers them something they want such as value, education, or entertainment. It is vital to understand what they want and need to create the right vehicle to get their attention. When they come upon content that is relevant to them or teaches them something of interest, the changes in engagement will blossom.

Six Ways to Go From Good to Great Content

1. Create content that has a consistent flow and feels authentic to the user.
2. Strive to cover the most important issues that are on the minds of your target audience (looking older or losing your hair).
3. Share what the impact of that issue may have on their lives in an empathetic way (self-esteem or loss of confidence).
4. Describe why patients may feel it is important (to feel better, compete in the workplace, mommy makeover).
5. Share the best outcomes of individual patients who were happy with the treatment plan or strategies you offered.
6. Offer alternative, less invasive, or expensive solutions (home care products or lifestyle adjustments).

A PLEA FOR DITCHING STOCK IMAGES

Let's face it – stock images are so 2015!

Time after time we see the same tired images of "pretty woman with long brown hair" or "woman in a bikini"plastered all over aesthetic practice websites and medspa marketing materials.

These same images pop up so much that I feel like they are my family, and I should invite them for Thanksgiving dinner!

Today, you can do much better. If you must use stock images, avoid the ones with a doctor or nurse with a stethoscope hung around their neck. The last time most aesthetic doctors used one was probably in residency.

Choose images that are appealing, realistic, and actually look a bit like your audience, so they can relate to them. Try to make them your own by changing the color palette, altering the background, or cropping them in a clever way so they can be uniquely your own.

I get that sometimes you need to pull some images for posters or eblasts – but there are so many better choices to tap into now. There is really no excuse anymore for using outdated images for your marketing with the popularity of Canva and other platforms. Make the image your own by manipulating it.

NEWS FLASH: AI platforms offer unlimited ways to create stunning unique images – so get going.

Ten Tools You Can Use for Images

1. Jumpstory.com – jumpstory.com
2. Pixabay – pixabay.com
3. Unsplash – unsplash.com
4. Pexels – pexels.com
5. Burst by Shopify – burst.shopify.com
6. Creative Market – creativemarket.com
7. Stocksnap – stocksnap.io
8. Gratisography – gratisography.com
9. Vistacreate – create.vista.com
10. PicJumbo – https://picjumbo.com

Consumer Engagement

Consumers are eager to engage with brands online, but they expect to get something in return for their time and attention.

You don't have to attract huge numbers of potential customers to be successful; you just need to attract the right ones. By casting the net wide enough to not miss anyone, you may be attracting people who are a waste of time and budget. The most important goal is to attract the right consumers who can become potential clients or patients or advocates. If you cast your marketing net too widely, you may waste time and money attracting the wrong consumers who are not interested in what you offer or live halfway across the world.

Strive to educate consumers on how you can meet and exceed their needs.

The most effective content can be generated by listening to your customers. Learn what they are interested in hearing from you, in what form, and how often. Educate patients' needs so they understand how they can benefit from need what you offer, what problem or concern you can solve for them, and feel confident that you can deliver their desired solution.

Customer-Friendly Marketing Strategies

To cut through all the clutter, tell a story that stands out and draws the reader in. Don't just focus on promoting your services and products, or tooting your own horn, but rather focus on your clients needs.

For example, what information would your ideal clients find valuable enough to want to learn more about?

Strive to resonate with potential clients who can visualize themselves having some of the services you offer as solutions to their goals. For example, when a potential customer reaches out after watching a video or listening to a podcast, they may refer to what encouraged them to learn more. This offers clues to learn how well your marketing strategy is working.

Because consumers are basically controlling the conversation, storytelling is always in demand. Storytelling, like the kind of content used on Instagram and Snapchat for example, allows potential patients to feel like they already know and trust you before they ever come to your practice.

The Value of Blogs

Although using video to reach your target audience is a hot commodity, don't overlook the value of strategic blog content. Blogs posted on your practice's website about interesting topics can help with SEO if you incorporate the requisite keywords. It can also establish your authority as an expert in your field.

In the scheme of things, blogs are also a relatively affordable type of platform for adding useful content to your site and can be repurposed for other consumer-facing channels, such as social media. They are a good strategy for adding timely content on key topics that will be of interest to your target audiences.

Blogging establishes authority and helps to generate traffic. Thus, incorporating these posts into a robust multipurpose marketing strategy offers numerous advantages. For example, well-written blogs rich with keywords can help to drive more traffic to your site.

You can reach out to your database and position your website as a valuable authority to answer their relevant queries and keep them updated on new trends, treatments, and interesting news.

Reinforce Your Expertise

Blogs can help establish your credentials and expertise with a wide range of readers who matter to your practice. Try to get a cadence going that is manageable, such as monthly or bi-weekly to start. This will help connect you with your audience on a steady basis to offer unique perspectives on topics that resonate with them.

Build your credibility by adding stats and studies to back up your point of view. You may consider inviting known industry experts or other professional colleagues to write about their perspectives on topics to keep your blog from becoming a one-note feature.

Always include some form of visuals, such as videos, infographics, images, or GIFs, to make the blog more eye-catching to your readers. Choose topics that are relevant to your current patients as well as target audiences. The blogs you post should be uniquely your own. You can outsource the writing to beauty and health writers or to competent SEO experts as needed.

Blogging can drive new traffic to your website since Google likes websites with updated and high-quality content. The amount of quality content on your website is a critical success factor in search engine indexing. You can post special events, offers, flash sales, and other announcements, but blogs should also have an educational tone. Be honest and sincere, rather than purely promotional. You can recommend products or services without appearing overtly salesy.

Caveat: Don't use free blogging platforms to host your content or lift content from other blogs without permission or credit. Google may punish you for these acts of laziness.

Blogging is still an ideal way of utilizing search engine optimization practices to help get your content noticed. By optimizing your website for search engines with interesting blog posts, your business will appear at the top of search results for topics related to the services you offer. This will lead to more visitors to your website, increase your leads, and help you grow your practice. You can post a blog with keywords weekly, but unless the content is valuable, you may lose your readers' interest. If you do not have time to draft quality blog posts on a regular basis, or if there is no one on your staff who can keep up with content creation, consider hiring a professional beauty or health writer.

Your blog can also help to funnel new patients and clients to specific pages on your website, which hopefully can drive more revenue to your practice, and it affords you another way to stay relevant with current clients. Focus on topics and themes that are trending and interesting to your audience.

Quality trumps quantity in all forms of content marketing. If you want your blogs to be read by the right audience, Keep your blogs and website copy interesting, informative, and teach them something they didn't know with each blog you post. Always add a visual in the form of a photo or video for best results.

Mastering the CTA

Calls-to-action (CTAs) are a tried and true lead generation strategy. In fact, all or most of your marketing tactics – social media updates, press releases, blog posts, eblasts, newsletters, and seminar invitations – will perform best when you include some form of CTA.

A CTA should appeal to your target audience so they will take the action you want them to take. For example, it should encourage them to do something, such as click, call, schedule, buy, etc. Your practice website should have a call-to-action also, in the form of a response you want users to complete. This can include filling out a contact form, signing up for a newsletter, or scheduling a consultation.

Active Urgent Language

A call-to-action should clearly tell users what you want them to do (Figure 5.2). It should include active words to compel users to act on your content:

- Buy.
- Call.
- Click.
- Enter to win.
- Go to.
- Register.

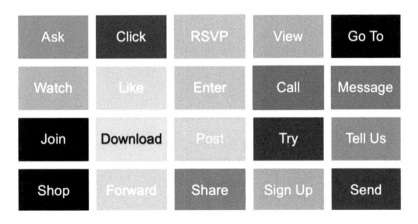

FIGURE 5.2 Words to use to encourage a reponse

- RSVP.
- Schedule.
- Share.
- Shop.
- Sign up.
- Subscribe.
- View

Take your CTA one step further by adding copy to encourage the user to act by a specific time, such as:

- *Offer expires April 30...*
- *For a short time only...*
- *Order now and receive a free gift...*
- *The first ten people who respond...*
- *Valid for 30 days...*
- *Space is limited...*
- *Last chance to save...*

Don't Hide Your CTA

If your CTA is positioned where there is a lot of other content or features to distract the viewer , they may get lost in the clutter. Post it where users are most likely to see it so they can act on it swiftly. Adding color can also be an effective way of gaining attention. The more prominent your call-to-action is, the greater the chance it will be noticed.

Using color is an effective way of drawing attention to specific elements, especially if the rest of the page is relatively neutral. The position, color, and white space surrounding your CTA are all keys to success.

Think about what happens when a user responds to your call-to-action. The rest of the process should be carefully thought out, so the back end is seamless, and the promised benefits are provided in a timely fashion.

Think of infomercials and home shopping networks that are well-versed in using CTAs brilliantly. Before they ask buyers to respond, they identify a problem and present a product that offers a solution. Then, there is a high degree of urgency created to get viewers to respond immediately "while supplies last." When the counter comes up and inventory is going fast, it prompts the viewer to grab one before it's too late.

How to Incentivize Your Target Audience

Clearly explain what the user will gain by taking the desired action. In some cases, you may add incentives to encourage users to complete a call-to-action. Consider the best way to communicate the benefits to the user, such as a benefit to those who sign up early or refer their friends and family.

Keep it simple by not having too many CTAs that may overwhelm the visitor who could get annoyed or confused and opt-out. Keep track of how many clicks it takes to act on the offer and consider how to streamline the process to get a better response.

All or most of the marketing tactics you use, including every page of your website, social media updates, press releases, blog posts, eblasts, newsletters, seminar invitations, etc., should include some form of CTA that leads the user to take action, such as click, call, schedule, buy, etc.

TYPES OF DIGITAL CONTENT

If you plan to work with creators or influencers, familiarize yourself with their lingo. Use the checklist here to consider the type of digital content you want for your marketing strategy in the forms of text, video, and images.

Text

- Articles.
- Blog Posts.
- Guides.
- Reviews.
- White Papers.
- E-books.
- Case Studies.
- Product Content.
- Captions.

Video

- Tutorials.
- Reviews.
- Vlogs (aka video blogs).
- Behind-the-scenes.
- Interviews.
- Webinars.
- Presentations (slides or decks).
- User-generated content (UGC).
- Contests.
- Giveaways.
- Livestreams.
- Q&As.

Images

- Photos.
- UGC.
- Infographics.
- Memes.
- GIFs.
- Quotes.
- Illustrations.

TOOLS YOU CAN USE

Note: Some offer a free vs. paid version.

Canva: For those of us who are not pros at Photoshop or InDesign, Canva is a godsend. This design program has become essential for businesses from small to huge. You can create branded images, social posts for all channels, brochures, and a zillion other things limited only by your creativity. Did I mention that the Canva app now features AI too? https://www.canva.com/

Creative Market: An online marketplace for community-generated design assets. The company sells fonts, graphics, illustrations, mockups, icons, templates, web themes, stock photography, and other digital goods for use by web creatives. https://creativemarket.com/

Copyscape: Copyscape provides a free plagiarism checker for finding copies of your web pages online, as well as two more powerful professional solutions for preventing content theft and content fraud. The software lets you detect duplicate content and check if your text is original. https://www.copyscape.com/

Google Alerts: Google Alerts is a free notification service provided by Google that sends emails to subscribers summarizing the search activity around selected search terms. https://www.google.com/alerts

Google Docs: Google Docs is a free cloud-based system that may be used to create documents or spreadsheets that can be edited and stored as part of the Google Docs Editors suite. This platform also features Google Sheets, Google Slides, Google Drawings, Google Forms, Google Sites, and Google Keep. https://www.google.com/docs

Grammarly: If auto-correct is your arch-enemy, Grammarly is the antidote. The software corrects your syntax and spelling as you are typing to avoid any snafus. It can call out anything from teeny grammatical errors as you are typing to more major mistakes that could be embarrassing if you don't catch them. It is a lifesaver. https://www.grammarly.com/

Otter.ai: Otter.ai uses AI to write automatic meeting notes with real-time transcription, recorded audio, automated slide capture, and automated meeting summaries. https://otter.ai/

Quillbot: Quillbot is an online writing assistant that uses AI and machine learning to paraphrase sentences. It boasts several tools used by millions of people worldwide who want to improve their writing. https://quillbot.com/

SemRush: SemRush is an all-in-one tool suite for improving online visibility and discovering marketing insights. Their tools and reports can help marketers that work in the following services: SEO, PPC, SMM, Keyword Research, Competitive Research, PR, Content Marketing, Marketing Insights, and Campaign Management. https://www.semrush.com/

Slack: Slack is a messaging app for businesses that connects people to the information they need. By bringing people together to work as one unified team, Slack transforms the way organizations communicate. https://slack.com/

WeTransfer: WeTransfer is a file transfer service that allows you to send large files over the internet. Using WeTransfer is very easy – upload your files, enter your email address, the email of the recipient, the WeTransfer verification code, and your files will be sent. https://wetransfer.com/

WORD TO THE WISE

In our fast-paced world, we all get bombarded with information in many forms from all directions on a minute-by-minute basis. Thus, the most effective content to accomplish your marketing goals should be uber-targeted, highly engaging, memorable, and platform-specific. Don't waste your readers' time – or they may never come back!

Mixing It Up

It can be a smart strategy to surprise your audience by sometimes mixing up your content. Try to avoid using the same formats too frequently or repeating themes and images unless they perform really well.

Consider using some of these content ideas to keep your audience engaged.

Social Media Content Checklist

- 5-star reviews and ratings.
- Behind-the-scenes.
- Blog posts.
- Case studies.
- Checklists.
- E-books.
- Employee appreciation.
- FAQs.
- How-to's.
- Information on procedures offered.
- Instagram stories and reels.
- Instagram threads.
- Interviews.
- Listicles.
- Patient journeys.
- Podcasts.
- Practice or medspa news.
- Press releases.
- Product recommendations.
- Question and answers.
- Quotes from key stakeholders.
- Resources page.
- Templates for office forms.
- Testimonials from happy patients.
- UGC.
- Video testimonials.
- Video tutorials.
- Webinars.
- Whitepapers.
- YouTube threads.

Social media users want quick, eye-catching, easy-to-read content to take in. But if an amazing and memorable photo catches their attention, they may share it with their followers.

The Scoop on LinkedIn

LinkedIn was once considered to be a safe place where professionals could congregate and share information.

I jumped on the original LinkedIn platform long before Microsoft picked it up. Since they acquired the platform in 2016, they have added a lot of clever features that have increased traffic exponentially. They have also made content more shareable and provided a user-friendly way to connect with colleagues, partners, industry professionals, influencers, creators, and more.

LinkedIn is widely considered a B2B (business to business) channel, yet many brands and individuals also use it for D2C (direct to consumer) communication and to elevate their personal and business platforms. This may include notices of open times for appointments, new treatments on offer, clinic news, etc.

There is nothing ostensibly wrong with this strategy, although I personally don't go there. I guess I am a LinkedIn veteran and a purist. I don't go on that platform to learn about anyone's birthday or what they did on their vacation. In fact, I personally find it annoying.

LinkedIn groups are also a powerful aspect of LinkedIn for connecting with like-minded individuals on a long list of important topics. Choose a topic and you will find numerous groups on relevant subjects, including dermatology, plastic surgery, aesthetic medicine, drugs, meetings, devices, injectables, and much more.

It is also a very useful site for finding partners and employees, following brands and companies you are interested in, and engaging with colleagues from all over the world.

SETTING UP A POWERFUL LINKEDIN PAGE

Make sure your brand's LinkedIn page is well-optimized and includes relevant and up-to-date information. Google ranks LinkedIn pages in search engines so optimizing your LinkedIn page should be a key piece of your marketing strategy and overall marketing efforts. According to LinkedIn, pages with complete information receive 30% more views than those that are incomplete.[*]

---

[*] https://www.hubspot.com/hubfs/How%20to%20Run%20Successful%20LinkedIn%20Ads%202023%20Update.pdf?li _fat_id=d6746e9a-5ef2-40d5-850b-3b12efbf6128.

6

Social Media Strategies Revisited

Content is fire; social media is gasoline.

Jay Baer, Entrepreneur and Best-Selling Author

Social media has morphed from being measured just by the number of followers a user attracts, to the quality of the content they post, and so much more.

Clearly, social media is one arena of marketing that has been in a constant state of flux all the way back to the first time we heard about it.

The Evolution of Social Media

Remember the first time you ever heard of this new entity called "social media"?

Take yourself all the way back to 1997. "Six Degrees" is credited with being the first platform to have launched a social media site in the format we know today. It enabled users to upload a profile and make friends with other users.[*]

I bet many people will remember Friendster, launched in 2002 and developed to be a dating site to help set up people with friends in common. That site tanked due to an overload of users that their services couldn't keep up with.

Next came Myspace, "a place for friends," in 2003 which quickly became the go-to site for teens. By 2005, the site had 25 million users.

Who, What, When? Social Media Milestones

- 2003 – LinkedIn, YouTube
- 2004 – Facebook
- 2005 – Reddit
- 2006 – Twitter
- 2007 – Tumblr, Hashtags were born
- 2010 – Instagram, Pinterest
- 2011 – Snapchat
- 2012 – Facebook acquires Instagram
- 2012 – Selfies were born
- 2013 – Vine, Slack
- 2016 – TikTok

Practically from its inception, we have been bombarded with constant changes and new platforms emerging daily, which necessitate keeping up with the trends to stay current and relevant.

---

[*] https://blog.hootsuite.com/history-social-media/

DOI: 10.1201/9780429356742-6

For what it's worth, my personal philosophy is not to be the first in my circle to jump into any new platform until it has been sufficiently vetted and proven its worth.

Time is money. Thus, I am reluctant to dive right into the next new channel until it gets vetted by more tech-savvy users than myself.

Here's why.

Where Are They Now

Remember when Meerkat and Periscope were at war for ownership of the live-streaming craze? We were told to go out and get the requisite equipment to get on board too.

A more recent example is clubhouse (with a small "c"). I was pressured by some colleagues to jump on this new platform that emerged in 2023. After spending a few months buying into their elitist game, I found that the amount of time required to invest in this platform totally unmanageable.

As so when many platforms start out, they are hot for a bit, and everyone jumps on. If they don't deliver on their promises of good content, simple user interface, and time vs. value ratio, people start to drop off.

The red flag with clubhouse was that it started out as an "invitation only" membership, which is a kind of cheesy strategy I tend to be leery of. You had to wait until someone invited you to join the site, which makes it seem very posh and exclusive. Another caveat was that you granted them access to your phone book! They also made it very tricky to get off their platform when you wanted to. This was a huge red flag. It was an elaborate scheme to keep their user numbers up and I wasn't having it!

So, is clubhouse still a thing? That seems to be unclear, as we have seen some apps rally after a disappointing performance. Considering the mass exodus of key stakeholders, the platform is in desperate need of getting acquired or having an influx of capital in order to go after more members.

After this experience, I am less inclined to jump on any new platform before it has been vetted by the pros. Thus, when BeReal popped up in 2020, I watched and waited to see where it would go. According to the site, https://bereal.com, BeReal has over 20 million daily active users around the world.

P.S. I don't know anyone in my circle who uses either of these sites anymore.

Channels and sites may come and go. But then again, whoever thought TikTok would rise to quick fame when it first entered the scene? So, it's a good idea to pay attention to the new ones coming out if they are geared towards the audience you want to reach.

Most social channels tend to catch the eye of early adopters, like Gen Z and Gen Y. Then some newbies will catch the eye of a wider range of users. Think about the rise of Instagram, for example.

Users per Channel and Gender Identification via Shopify (as of 2023)

- Facebook: 2.93 billion users – 56% male/44% female
- YouTube: 2.52 billion users – 53.6% male/46% female
- WhatsApp: 2 billion users – 54% male/46% female
- Instagram: 1.39 billion users – 44% male/55.6% female
- WeChat: 1.3 billion users – 64.3% male/35.7% female
- Messenger: 976 million users – 55.5% male/44.5% female
- TikTok: 945 million users – 40% male/60% female
- Telegram: 700 million users - 58.6% male/41.4% female
- Douyin: 613 million users – 55% male/45% female (China)
- Snapchat: 293 million users – 44.6% male/54.4% female
- QQ Messenger: 574 million users – 52.3% male/47.7% female (China)
- VKontakte: 49% male/51% female (Russia & Eastern Europe)

Source: shopify.com/blog/most-popular-social-media-platforms

THE SCOOP ON TIKTOK (AS OF THIS PRINTING)

1. *TikTok will reach 1.8 billion users by the end of 2023.*
2. *It is on fire in many locations around the world – both in terms of its ever-expanding user base as well as the amount of content that is generated daily.*
3. *The majority of TikTok users are under 30, with the largest age bracket between 20 and 29 years old.*
4. *TikTok is used by more women than men, but that gap is closing.*
5. *Outside of China, TikTok's largest markets are the US, Indonesia, and Brazil.*
6. *On average, US adult users spend 33 minutes per day on TikTok, ranking it second by daily engagement after Facebook with 35 minutes (users on both platforms are basically equivalent).*

Sources: https://backlinko.com/tiktok-users#monthly-active-tiktok-users;
https://www.businessofapps.com/data/tik-tok-statistics/

Fourteen Government TikTok Bans

To date, TikTok is active in over 150 countries.
Most common reasons for a TikTok ban? Cybersecurity concerns.

1. Afghanistan: Taliban leadership banned TikTok on the grounds of protecting young people from "being misled."
2. Australia: TikTok was banned from devices issued by the Australian federal government.
3. Belgium: Belgium temporarily banned TikTok from devices owned or paid for by the federal government, citing worries about cybersecurity, privacy, and misinformation.
4. Canada: Canada announced that government-issued devices must not use TikTok, and employees will also be blocked from downloading the app in the future.
5. Denmark: Denmark's Defense Ministry banned its employees from having TikTok on their work phones, ordering staffers who have installed it to remove the app as soon as possible.
6. European Union: The European Parliament, European Commission, and the EU Council imposed a TikTok ban on staff devices, and lawmakers and staff were advised to remove the app from their personal devices.
7. France: "Recreational" use of TikTok and other apps like Twitter and Instagram on government employees' phones is banned. The French government noted the decision came after other governments took measures targeting TikTok.
8. India: A nationwide ban imposed on TikTok and many other Chinese apps like WeChat over privacy and security concerns was made permanent in January 2021.
9. Latvia: The app is prohibited from official foreign ministry smartphones.
10. Netherlands: The Dutch government banned apps including TikTok from employee work phones, citing data security concerns.
11. New Zealand: Government officials are prohibited from having the app on their work phones, following advice from government cybersecurity experts.
12. Norway: Norwegian parliament banned TikTok on work devices for government officials.
13. Pakistan: Pakistani authorities temporarily banned TikTok at least four times since 2020, citing concerns over immoral content.

14. Taiwan: Government devices, including mobile phones, tablets, and desktop computers, are not allowed to use Chinese-made software including Doyin (TikTok) or Xiaohongshu, a Chinese lifestyle content app.

Source: https://apnews.com/article/tiktok-ban-privacy-cybersecurity-
bytedance-china-2dce297f0aed056efe53309bbcd44a04

The Clock is TikTok-ing

The frenzy around TikTok started in 2018 when it merged with its parent company Byte Dance's musical .ly platform, and it continues to skyrocket. The app is the self-proclaimed leading destination for short-form mobile video.

The platform has undoubtedly made an unprecedented impact on social media trends and pop culture in many countries around the world.

At least in part, TikTok has focused on targeting businesses, creating more options for advertising, and expanding into a platform that brands want to be active on because it delivers results for their campaigns. The app has grown by leaps and bounds in terms of brand awareness despite being banned in some countries.

They have made a significant play to deliver tools for businesses and to improve the way the platform can be optimized for social selling and customer engagement. Growing brand awareness on the app requires more of a focus on social media than lead generation.

Welcome TikTok Creators

It can be challenging and exhausting for many brands to create content that consistently engages consumers across multiple channels. This is where creators have found their niche.

"Content creator" is a very popular and desirable job description. It has become a cottage industry, perhaps more so due to TikTok's speedy rise than any other platform. This is where content creators seem to have originated, and they are not to be confused with high-level influencers. Creators can include freelancers, customers, experts in a niche area, and all sorts of individuals. This pushes brands to invest in influencers and content creators to take their content to the next level.

TikTok is also very focused on creating opportunities for their top-tier users (i.e., creators, brands, agencies) and generating additional revenue for them. They are very prolific at working with these mega clients. Like Meta, gaming is a big priority and there is a focus on creating an environment that is user-friendly to entice more gamers.

As TikTok continues to evolve and dominate the social landscape, there are some caveats to keep in mind. For example, are you just generating awareness, or are you seeing new paying clients coming to your practice directly from this app?

While both can be good for your business, random awareness among a demographic that is not interested in or cannot afford to have exclusive and pricey treatments or buy products probably won't do much for your bottom line.

TikTok Trends

More than any other social platform, TikTok can be as addictive as chocolate.

According to Influencer Marketing Hub:

* It is the most popular app downloaded globally.
* On average, users spend more than 1.5 hours per day on TikTok.
* Highest social media engagement rates per post.

- More women use TikTok than men in most markets.
- Most popular relevant categories overall include entertainment, dance, fitness/sports, beauty/skincare, fashion, and cooking.
- Gets significantly more engagement than Instagram and YouTube.

Eight Hot TikTok Trends To Know About For An Aesthetic Practice

1. TikTok Made Me Buy It: This indicates that you have bought a product that went viral on the app when influencers and creators shared their thoughts about items.
2. TikTok Voice Effects: Voice changer feature that you can use to modify the sound of your voice in videos.
3. TikTok Now: A way to be entertained and connect with other users.
4. TikTok Fitness: All about fitness goals, workout routines, and staying healthy. Hashtag #fittok has a few hundred million views.
5. TikTok Skincare: The newest platform of choice for skincare routines and product recommendations from consumers, dermatologists, medspas, etc.
6. TikTok Selfcare: Users share their favorite selfcare practices which can be anything from spa treatments to home care pampering.
7. TikTok Drop Shipping: This is just what you think. It is a way to sell products by either shipping directly to clients or through a manufacturer that will ship merchandise from a warehouse.
8. TikTok Makeup: Another way to promote cosmetics through the app where users go for recommendations and can make a purchase instantly.

TikTok, like Meta, is highly focused on monetizing the platform, so many of their new launches will have that in mind. They recently created a shop in the US, and the site also launched an ad revenue-sharing plan for their top creators.

Many of the trends on TikTok can turn into the most popular trends on online, so it is wise to follow these trends even if you are not very active on the channel.

TikTok is now at a stage that makes it truly too big to fail. In fact, there have been organized protests online to deter any thoughts of banning or restricting the site in the future. In this uncertain economy, restricting the livelihoods of creators and brands would result in riots in the streets, at least in the US market.

As much as the old geezers in the US Congress, who can't even pronounce "TikTok", would love to ban this uber-popular global site because it is owned by a Chinese company, it is doubtful that this will ever happen. TikTok is highly profitable and individuals as well as business users are big fans.

"Remember That Time Is Money"

Benjamin Franklin penned this classic phrase which first appeared in an essay, "Advice to a Young Tradesman," for a book chapter he wrote in 1748, almost three centuries ago. Yet, this is as true today as when Ben picked up his quill to write it.

I keep this phrase in the back of my mind whenever I find myself performing a random task that could easily be delegated or automated, or when my team gets bogged down by workloads that a bot could cut through in half the time.

This understanding relies on automation tools for internal processes and to enhance customer experience. These include marketing tools for CRM (customer relationship management), social media, advertising, lead management, and emails.

Anything that can help you save time and enhance productivity is a big plus. Keep your eyes out for the plethora of new launches and next-level tools to help simplify automation and personalization.

For example, if there is a task that you would be eager to streamline or simplify, chances are there's an app for that.

Social media users continue to skyrocket, which has a lot to do with the day-to-day rise of new and exciting platforms, better content solutions, and automation tools that are making social channels slightly easier to handle. "Slightly" is the operative word.

The social channels that will be most important for your aesthetic practice or medspa will vary significantly by market. You will have to review each channel that your current patients are most active on and that are most important to them.

According to Hootsuite the average user will visit 7.2 social media platforms each month.

TWENTY TOP RATED SOCIAL MEDIA MARKETING TOOLS*

1. Social Champ.
2. Social Status.
3. eClincher.
4. SocialPilot.
5. Visme.
6. SociAlert.
7. CoSchedule.
8. Sendible.
9. Statusbrew.
10. Tailwind.
11. Post Planner.
12. Postfity.
13. Loomly.
14. Zoho Social.
15. Social Insider.
16. Radaar.
17. Metricool.
18. OkToPost.
19. Vistacreate.
20. QRTiger.

* See further: https://buffer.com/library/social-media-management-tools/; https://blog.hootsuite.com/social-media-scheduling-tools/; https://sproutsocial.com/insights/

Most practices cannot stretch their staff or budget to be everywhere effectively, so they must narrow down the list. It is more prudent to be active and effective on a handful of the most relevant channels than to try to be everywhere in a less effective way.

Evaluate your performance on each channel and confirm that your key target audiences are active and engaged. If you don't have the bandwidth to grow the channels effectively while staying on brand, you may not be effective. This cancels out any potential value it may have yielded.

Social media is a two-way dialogue.

FIVE WAYS TO ENGAGE WITH YOUR FOLLOWERS

1. *Stimulate a conversation in a "true or false?" format.*
2. *Poll your followers: "What's your favorite?" This could be a skincare product, facial treatment, lip filler, toxin, body shaping device, etc.*
3. *Introduce each staff member by name with a candid photo, their position, and something personal so patients can get familiar with your team.*
4. *Highlight and tag any charitable organizations or causes you support.*
5. *Try some "Test your knowledge" posts such as, "What's the most popular lip filler?" or "What is PRP?"*

Instagram Reels

Reels is Meta's answer to TikTok. Reels are short-form Instagram videos that can be up to 90 seconds long. Users can record, edit, and clip videos and photos together, set them to music, and post to their feed.

Since this feature turned up, Instagram Reels has been on fire and is considered the most used feature on IG for many dedicated users. It has also benefitted creators and influencers by extending the ability to monetize their Reels.

Instagram Live

Instagram Live can be used to do live chats, interviews, or how-to virtual events through your IG channel. These are easy to do and last up to one hour, when IG cuts you off. Most lives go for around 30 minutes because the average person's attention span keeps shrinking.

Try a series of Instagram Lives on key topics of interest to stay engaged with your fans and followers. Increase your mobile website-based advertising to reach them and utilize a text messaging program for specials and promotions. Keep in mind that most consumers are more likely to shop when they are relaxed and not under stress.

Setting a Budget

I added this spreadsheet model to underscore the fact that social media is not free.

If you don't believe me, just ask Mark Zuckerberg. The users you see online, who are not supermodels or athletes, that have hundreds of thousands of followers, pristine images, gorgeous glamour shots, etc. are investing in their digital profile. In most cases, it is paying off.

More is more when it comes to digital marketing. But the benefits are that your activity is trackable, so you can measure your success and manage it carefully through the available analytics. You can't really do that with print, radio, or TV spots.

So, I have included a list of the expenses that will arise when executing a proper social media strategy. You can fill in the frequency and cost per task to get your budgeting straight (Figure 6.1).

Caveat: *Most apps are free or charge a nominal fee for basic usage. Beware that many of them include additional hidden costs to grant access to advanced features.*

When it comes to taking great photos for your marketing, the tools you use count.

If you are fortunate to have someone on staff who takes great photos and videos, you are truly blessed. It is a very helpful skill to have on board.

However, there are some great tools and apps available that will make it much easier to generate professional-looking content, even for novices.

TACTIC	FREQUENCY	COSTS	TOTAL
CONTENT CREATION			
DASHBOARD PLATFORM			
PHOTOS/IMAGES			
PROMOTIONS / GIVEAWAYS			
CONTENT CREATORS			
VIRTUAL EVENTS			
EQUIPMENT			
INFLUENCERS			
SOCIAL ADS			
EXTERNAL VENDORS			
APPS			

FIGURE 6.1   Budgeting for Social Media Marketing

Start with a current high-quality iPhone (or Android) that has a top-of-the-line camera. Your phone or tablet can basically replace an SLR camera for most of the social content you will need.

Then choose some easy-to-use apps that can take your pics and videos to the next level in terms of filters, lighting, cropping, and editing. There is an infinite selection to choose from wherever you get your apps.

Tools You Can Use

Here are a dozen popular tools to check out. These were hand-picked by my team for their ease of use, problem-solving, and affordability – most are free or cheap to use.

Caveat: Draft a formal policy clarifying the rules for all staff members on posting about clinic patients on their own channels, and have all staff sign the document.

Look into an External Agency

An external agency could be a marketing communications firm like mine or your web or SEO team. The fees may be worth it to take your social to the next level and relieve your staff of some of the heavy lifting and time-consuming work. Ask for references to be sure you have the right team before committing to a contract.

What about Bringing on a Freelancer?

Enlisting a freelancer can work for many practices. However, it can be somewhat risky. A member of the practice will need to manage external teams carefully. At the end of the day, your license is on the line.

In this case, direct instructions need to be shared in writing and all content should be approved before it gets posted to stay safe. The best way to facilitate this is by using a dashboard platform so whoever is managing this process in the practice can approve all content before it gets posted. That is how my social team works with brands and practices.

Maybe a College Student?

Although I recognize that this may seem like a reasonable idea, it may present challenges due to exams and other commitments that may limit the time available for training and nurturing students to run your social for a patient-focused business.

Maybe a College Intern?

Depending on the age and education of the intern, this can be a little risky and will require a lot of supervision, which may defeat the advantage of having someone help with social.

What about Enlisting a Family Member?

This can easily be a disaster depending on the situation and the relationship. In essence, keep in mind that it is hard to fire a relative.

Last but surely not least...

How Can AI Help with My Social Channels

Be honest. You are all thinking, "Hmmm how can we outsource some of these tedious bits of social to a robot?" It's a natural query. AI tools can absolutely help with content creation, both visual and text, plus social media monitoring. You may also take it to the next level by using AI to do the leg work for managing ads, identifying influencers or creators that are on brand for your business, and helping to promote campaigns to elevate brand awareness.

Bottom line: *A hybrid of some of the above-listed strategies may also be a good option. Do the simple tasks in-house and outsource what you don't have the time or expertise to do consistently.*

See further the social media manager job description in the Appendix.

Most Important Metrics and KPIs

Paying close attention to your metrics and KPIs (Key Performance Indicator) is crucial for determining how well your social is performing. Without measuring results, you may not be able to stay on course. These metrics are a critical success factor to help you hit your goals.

Four Metrics to Keep Tabs On

1. **Clicks**: This is the number of times consumers have clicked on your content. If you're able to identify what brings in clicks, you can replicate it.
2. **Engagement**: Engagement is defined as any interaction your audience has with your content. This helps you know how your audience perceives your brand and how eager they are for your content.
3. **Reach**: This is the number of unique users who have seen, but not necessarily interacted with, your post on their feeds.
4. **Hashtag performance**: This metric will help you determine what hashtags related to your brand are used by the most people in your audience.

Posting Cadence

One of the great debates of social media is how often you should post. There is no definitive answer to this, and it will vary considerably from business to business. Check out these guidelines to consider what will work best for your business and what your staff has the bandwidth to keep up with.

Social Media Reality Check

1. More is not necessarily more on social.
2. Quality trumps quantity.
3. All or most social networks are ad platforms, just like Google. So, you will need to have a budget to make big things happen, unless your last name is Kardashian.
4. Try posting less often and boosting your best posts more often and for longer to determine if that gives you better reach.
5. Most users don't want to see your content multiple times daily and maybe not even once a day. Space out your best content and keep them eager for more like that.

*Caveat: Buying fans and followers is a waste of time and money, and could ultimately damage your brand, growing your Instagram following with users in their teens from halfway across the world who never ever going to become actual patients will not help achieve your goals. **Don't buy followers – period!***

Ten Tips for Posting Best Practices

1. Post the right content on the right channel at the right time and get in a steady flow of posts for the best results.
2. Create more of the style and type of content that is performing best for each of your channels.
3. Boost the most valuable content with promotions on Facebook, Instagram, TikTok, WhatsApp, or Snapchat depending on the most popular channels you are active on.
4. Monitor results closely – engagement is the key metric.
5. Prioritize Instagram as the hero platform in relevant markets, like the US. Choose another channel that moves the needle for you in other markets.
6. In terms of IG Lives, stories, story highlights, reels, polls, quizzes, and short-form videos, if they generate traction, try it again. If they fall flat, either rethink your method or abandon them.
7. Activate social shopping so consumers can purchase products and services from their phones and social apps seamlessly (if this is allowed in your market).
8. Position your brand as an authority and resource by featuring expert commentary and educational content on your channels.
9. Include images of diversity – skin tones, ethnicities, genders, age groups, treatments, etc.
10. Leverage paid media to drive reach and help to grow a strong, loyal following.

Using the right tone for your content and consistency will make your channels more professional and polished, which speaks to who you are as a practitioner and business leader. Make sure that your social is always on brand for your practice and persona. If you deviate too much, your brand may suffer.

Caveat: Keep your medical license in mind and comply with all healthcare regulations and privacy rules in your market. You are responsible for your license – not your staff or an external agency.

THINK BEFORE POSTING

Ask yourself, do I really want to share this with my followers?
If you're not sure, ask your team and make sure they understand that you really want an honest response, which is what I do, so they can be straight with you. If my team doesn't recommend that I post certain content, even if I think it is brilliant, I do not hesitate to drop it. It's okay to go with your instincts, but getting a second opinion is always a helpful reality check. Listen to your trusted team who (hopefully) has your best interests at heart.

Strategies for Social Success

More brands are entering the social media sphere daily as the average consumer's attention span keeps dwindling. There is steep competition for getting more eyes on your content. Thus, just creating entertaining content is not enough to reach your target audience and keep them engaged anymore.

Your content strategy should communicate with your audience in a meaningful way to keep them interested and coming back for more. Ideally, the optimal goal is to encourage your clients to share your best content with their friends so they will hopefully follow your channels too.

There is no "one-size-fits-all" secret to nailing a successful social media strategy, but there are some basics to guide you.

Always stay true to your brand, and that includes on your social channels. Don't risk undermining what you have worked so hard to build over time.

Start with a Plan

The importance of having a strategy for your brand cannot be overstated. Trying to copy strategies and content from big brands is a bad idea. These methods are not typically suited to small brands like a solo medical practice and tend to target bigger goals and objectives with huge budgets to get there.

Set out reasonable goals that are achievable. Every social media strategy starts with goals. Having distinct goals helps to identify what you want to achieve on social media within a specific period.

What to Know Before Launching a Social Media Campaign

How can we increase brand awareness?

Increasing brand awareness is the process of fostering familiarity between social media consumers and your product. This is a great goal if you're just starting out or announcing a new product.

How can we boost engagement?

If you notice that you aren't getting as much traction or as many likes as you used to, boosting engagement should be your top priority. Common ways to increase engagement include asking questions and creating interactive content. Think of videos as a preferred format of content.

How can we drive traffic to our website?

Social media is a great way to drive traffic to your site. Social media ads are like search engine ads and can be targeted and tracked to measure ROI.

Know your audience?

Don't make assumptions about their behavior and preferences. Use the right tools to help you analyze your target demographic. And if you're still not sure, just ask them. Active social users don't tend to be shy about voicing their opinions. In fact, some may be flattered that you are asking them and will share some good intel you can use.

Most Valuable Platforms

Marketers are tasked with creating a social media strategy that connects with consumers across generations. Each generation holds unique values, experiences, and behaviors that influence the content users create to attract them.

For example, beauty brands strive to catch the attention of Gen Z makeup lovers while speaking to Gen X about the age-reversing products they want. Understanding the differences and motivations behind each group of your patients, as well as the target audience you are trying to attract, is an important step to building trust.

Once you have zeroed in on whom you want to reach with each initiative, develop a marketing strategy that appeals to each of those target groups.

Almost every generation uses social media on a pretty regular basis, but the channels they flock to and the ways they use them are the points of difference.

I sometimes see octogenarians in airports or when I take my dog for a walk in Central Park who are fiddling with their tablets to connect with their grandchildren or to get information.

Powerful channels like Facebook and Instagram are ideal for intergenerational marketing tactics because they cast the widest net. This speaks to the value of a cross-channel social strategy that hits the mark with each of your target demographics. Intergenerational marketing can expand your audience and help you grow your community.

Speaking to consumers at different points along their lifespans commands a social strategy that spans age groups and demographics. Establishing unique content pillars is a critical success factor to engage each of your target audiences in a unique way.

Most Popular Channels by Demographic (Figure 6.2)

Facebook is still popular among Gen X and baby boomers, which may signal that it is the channel where brands go to target 45 to 80-year-olds, but this is very market dependent.

Only a relatively small portion of Gen Z use Facebook on a regular basis. Millennials were at the forefront of the rise of social media, and they are more likely to spend time across a wider range of platforms than prior generations. Unlike their younger counterparts, millennials have stayed true to channels like Instagram, TikTok, and Snapchat in some markets.

Gen Z is one of the most highly sought-after generations online and among the most complex. The first generation born in the digital age has unsurprisingly transformed the social media landscape. Gen Z is quick to jump on the latest channels and stay ahead of the trends. These users are also quick to follow the newest trends and stay abreast of the channels that are trending.

Posting Patient Photos

Every social media platform has rules and regulations about what you will be allowed to post. For example, Facebook and Instagram often remove or block posts with any kind of nudity or exaggerated

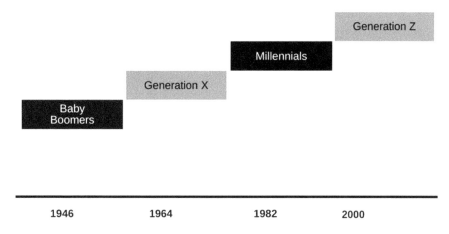

FIGURE 6.2   Generations Cheat Sheet

claims, sexual or intimate wellness messaging, and other terms that may get flagged. This tends to be very random. Some users will protest to get their copy to go live, but success is often sporadic because you will basically be pleading with a bot.

Caveat: In some markets, posting patient photos is not permitted at all or there are some restrictions. Check with your local medical council or relevant body in your area to learn precisely what you can and cannot do in your specific market. Be mindful of always getting written patient consent to post, repost, regram, etc. to be kept on file indefinitely. Patient photos are safest when used on organic posts, especially if the patient is identifiable, rather than on sponsored content. Monitor these posts to be sure your patients' images are not lifted from your channels to wind up on another clinic's marketing.

Alternative Ways to Use Patient Photos

In some markets, using real patients' photos on social channels or your website may be discouraged or can even be considered a patient confidentiality breach. This may present a challenge for many practitioners.

Having superior patient photographs, which are clearly labeled and taken at the same angle and sizing, speaks volumes for the results you can achieve.

Photos are what consumers are most interested in looking at on your website and social. They want to see what you do and visualize what can be achieved if they become your patient.

I recognize that this is a very controversial issue globally. Many practices are at a disadvantage in markets that enforce strict rules about sharing patient photos and may restrict any use of before-and-after images.

There are some workarounds to consider. One method I have come across is to use a patient video speaking about their experience after having a treatment. In this way, you may be able to share a "patient experience" that is not seemingly promising any specific outcomes.

KEEPING PATIENT PHOTOS SAFE

For aesthetic practitioners, your results are your calling card. But the regulations that govern how patient photographs should be stored and used by healthcare professionals vary by market.

Think of it this way. Basically, anything posted in a public forum is subject to being copied or exploited. To protect yourself and your patients, make it hard if not impossible for anyone to copy or share patient photos you share on your website and social channels.

Before you show or post any patient photos, you should be sure to have a written agreement from the patient to be kept on file that grants their permission to share, repost, or regram any images to your social channels or website. If the patient changes his or her mind at any time, it is their right to ask you to take it down.

Here are some viable tactics to protect your photos online:

- Add your own watermark positioned to deter anyone from cropping around them, such as your practice logo.
- Avoid posting high-resolution images – low resolution does not copy well.
- Review the terms of the websites you upload any patient photos to.
- Disable right clicks on the image wherever possible.
- Frame your image and include copyright details.
- Investigate sites that will track where your photos end up.

If you do find that your patient's photos have been lifted, rather than seek legal action, start by reaching out directly to the owner of the site or social channel to request that the photos be removed. They may not even be aware and will hopefully just take it down.

Value of Sharing Real Patient Photos

- Good photos sell more services and treatments – in fact, patient photos are known to be the aspect of practice websites that get the most traffic.
- You may start out with photos from companies you do business with when you are launching a new treatment or device and building up your own portfolio from there.
- Display results of what you can achieve with the treatments you do most frequently, if possible.
- Build up a portfolio of before-and-after photos of various conditions, skin types, ages, genders, and combination therapies.
- A bulletproof consent signed by your patient should be mandatory before sharing any patient photos.

The Ultimate Endorsement

Another strategy I recommend is sharing a video of aesthetic practitioners having one of the treatments they offer themselves. This strategy can be very effective, especially when you are introducing a new treatment. It can serve as a great way to instill confidence in your target audience by showing you are keen to have it done yourself. It is also great content for sharing.

This strategy makes patients feel at ease about how the treatment is performed when they see the practitioner experiencing it personally. At the same time, it offers a glimpse into the practitioner's personality.

- Photos/videos of practitioners having treatments ring true with consumers.
- Reinforces your confidence in the treatments you offer – being a patient yourself.
- Makes patients feel more comfortable about having a first-time procedure.

Try this strategy and monitor your engagement. I predict that it will perform well for you.

The best social media goal for attracting new patients: "I felt like I knew them before I visited the clinic..."

Content Themes

A content theme is a plan that helps you decide what to post in the long run and to create timely and thoughtful content.

Campaigns, products, storytelling, and partnerships are often top of mind when you're mapping out content pillars for your brand. While demographics and age groups come into play in larger marketing strategy sessions, they should also be part of your regular content-planning conversations. Once you nail down your target audiences, learn what styles and visuals resonate best with each audience to take your strategy to the next level.

Text-based content works well for reaching Facebook's most active users – baby boomers and Gen X. They go to Facebook to communicate with friends and family, and get information in the form of news, politics, lifestyle, and shopping. Serving your Facebook audience shareable content can increase your chances of conversion and greatly amplify your reach.

Millennials head to social media for community, discovery, and inspiration. While Instagram and TikTok are often their channels of choice, diversifying your social media approach will help to capture the attention of younger audiences. This generation is heavily influenced by their peers and online communities. They follow influencers and respond to community-created or user-generated content. They are also at the forefront of online shopping.

Leverage the right kind of timely content that resonates with millennials across all social platforms to maximize engagement. This generation has a short attention span and tends to be more fickle and less loyal than their older counterparts. So, if you don't meet their standards, you may lose them very quickly.

Use a Content Calendar

Create a monthly social content and marketing calendar to keep all your programs coordinated. The whole team needs to know what is happening when, why, and on what platforms, from a blog post to paid ads, e-blasts, events, and special offers for the month.

Social media doesn't stop on Friday at 6 PM when you close your clinic for the weekend. It is a 24/7, 365 days per year activity, so someone needs to be minding it all the time. This can be easily accomplished via text message notifications for comments, posts, and inquiries as they come in.

Social Media Management Platforms

If you are managing multiple channels, consider engaging a proper social media dashboard to work off.

These tools provide critical information you need to organize your channels, curate content, scheduling, and measure your performance. It can keep you updated on how you are doing so you can pivot your strategy if the results are not what you were aiming for.

For marketing managers, this is an essential tool for staying on top of the content being put out there, seeing how your team responds to it, and helping determine when to act.

These tools can be especially important if you are outsourcing your social content creation and posting. Ideally, you can be able to check, approve, or edit all content that goes out there in advance, organized in one easy-to-use dashboard.

It is a worthwhile expense that in turn will save you money by organizing what you need to follow in one easily accessible location. It will get the marketing team organized around the most critical KPIs and monitor how your social media activities are performing, and share the metrics about your followers and what the world is saying about you.

Five Reasons Why You Need a Dashboard

1. An essential tool to manage all or most channels in one organized spreadsheet format.
2. Free or paid versions are available with numerous helpful features to tap into including posts, replies, reposts, analytics, and custom reports.
3. Onsite and remote teams of users can work simultaneously.
4. Shares a day-to-day picture of your most important KPIs and how your social is performing.
5. Useful for social listening and following what people are saying about your brand.

EIGHT POPULAR SOCIAL MEDIA DASHBOARDS

Each market has options for free or paid subscriptions to tap into.
These are some of the best ones in the US

1. Buffer
2. Hootsuite
3. Sprout
4. Information Design
5. Later
6. Sendible
7. SocialBee
8. Agorapulse

Hashtag Strategy

Determine how you want to use hashtags. They can be used on all social channels except Snapchat. You can post a hashtag on Snapchat if you want to, but it won't be clickable or searchable.

The main use of hashtags is to help get your content found by users who are the most likely to be interested in what you post. This may include information about your practice, products, services, staff, and much more.

Hashtags can make your posts more discoverable. Add your location so your business can be found, and tag partners if you want to invite them to the conversation.

Keep them short, as in up to 12 characters and maximum 3 words. Any longer may be too hard to read. Instagram allows up to 24 characters.

Divide hashtags into relevant categories:

- **Ownable/Branded** (uniquely yours) – #DrWiseSays, #CornwallClinic, #AskMeAnything.
- **Product/Service/Treatment** – (what you offer or want to promote) #Laserhairremoval, #Microdermabrasion, #Lipfillers.
- **Industry Niche** (specific to what you do) – #Rhinoplastyexperts, #Skincarespecialists, #BestInjector.
- **Campaigns** (special offers, new treatments) – #FillerFriday, #ThrowbackThursday, #Holiday.
- **Promotions** (events, themes) – #SkincareSaturday, #TransformationTuesday.
- **Location** (target users around your location) – #ManhattanMedSpa, #SanFranFacialists, #TennesseeTattooRemoval.
- **Holidays/Special Dates** – #InternationalWomensDay, #SkinCancerAwareness, #GivingTuesday.

Rules of the Road for Great Collaborations

If you are collaborating with another business, brand, influencer, or hosting an event, create an ownable and unique hashtag specific to that collaboration to gain traction. Make it catchy, relevant, and clever to put a smile on the target audience's faces. Humor, creativity, and originality are also well-received.

- Check out any hashtags you are considering to be sure that no one has used them before you, or that there isn't some nefarious meaning to them you weren't aware of. Oops.
- Keep the hashtag short so people will remember it and use it without needing to look it up.
- It should be relevant to the campaign, the brands involved, and the mission so fans will use it in their posts.
- Encourage and incentivize people to use the hashtag to spread the word about your collaboration or event.
- Add keywords to make it searchable.

INSTA HASHTAGS
Instagram allows up to 30 hashtags per post
- *Don't feel that you must use 30 on every post!*
- *More is not necessarily more.*
- *Use the most relevant hashtags first.*

To find relevant hashtags, join conversations, and increase your footprint
- *Search for the hashtag on Instagram.*
- *Click on "Follow" to find out how popular it is.*

Caveat: Look out for "bashtags" – hashtags that have a negative connotation or a meaning you may not realize. Check it out before posting on ritetag.com, flick.com, or hashtagpicker.com

Newsflash: You Can't Really "Own" Your Followers

Why not?

Because if Meta shuts your Facebook or Instagram for whatever reason, they may take all your hard-earned fans and followers with them.

You may be able to get your channel back with followers, but what if you can't?

They could be gone forever, and we know how hard and expensive it is to start over from scratch.

How can you protect yourself?

By converting as many of your fans and followers to your own practice database. Once you have their contact details (phone, email, address), they can be yours forever.

Ad Strategies

Think about how many emails and ads flood your mailbox every day. Then factor in Gmail ads, Facebook ads, Instagram promotions, text messaging marketing, and automated calls to your mobile phone.

If you're like me, you want to scream. Sometimes when I hear a ding, I can't even figure out which device or platform it's coming from!

Consumers are bombarded with brands that are constantly sending them thousands of pieces of useless information. Most of the time, the content they get is not very relevant or useful, or it's just spam. This increased competition is forcing practitioners to reconsider what they are putting out there.

Therefore, make sure that every single post you publish has value for your target audience. The more targeted your content is, the better it will work for you. Targeted content sent to the right customer at the right time is the most effective at driving traffic and interest to your practice.

With the realization that consumers don't want to read random, impersonal content, the need to devise new ways of providing more engaging content to maintain your audience's attention is obvious.

Branded content does not need to be restricted for use on social media, blogs, and websites. Some of the most popular strategies include using branded blog posts, infographics, GIFs, videos, and other forms of content to reach audiences.

Working with Influencers and Creators

If you want to be Insta-famous, working with influencers can help to drive traction for your clinic, company, or product by promoting you to their fan base.

"Influencers" can be anyone with a robust following on Instagram, TikTok, YouTube, or another channel relevant to your business.

Eight Things to Look for with Influencers

1. Age appropriate *(Over 21 at minimum, mature enough to have credibility).*
2. Relatable to your patients.
3. Aspirational image and persona.
4. On brand with your practice values and positioning.
5. High engagement with followers.
6. Knowledgeable about aesthetic treatments, skincare, beauty products, etc.
7. Fans and followers are local to your business *(i.e., not based in Southeast Asia if your practice is located in Devon or Vancouver).*
8. Check for fake followers.

Search for local influencers who are on brand for your practice and match your target audience. Evaluate their image, content, post quality, tone, and style. Check out how they dress in posts and if there are spelling errors in their content.

Look at other collaborations they have done with brands. Check out what other products and brands they represent. If the influencer posts about having a lot of freebie aesthetic treatments from other clinics near you, it is probably best to move on. If they represent competitive practices or med spas, they may lose credibility with followers.

Most importantly, check how they identify "paid posts" in their feed. Every market has specific rules that apply to paid social media collaborations, and in some markets, such as the UK, France, the US, and others, fines can occur if you and/or the influencers are not in compliance.

These are six of the phrases and hashtags commonly used in English-speaking markets for posts that begin with something like *"I partnered with XYZ Klinik…"* or hashtags only may suffice.

1. #paidcollaboration
2. #paidpartnership
3. #paidsponsorship
4. #sponsored
5. #gifted
6. #affiliate

Instagram has a special feature where you can show a "paid partnership" by including a @ on your posts.

Caveat*: Check out the rules from the US Federal Trade Commission (FTC) on disclosures. They state that, "Truth in advertising is important in all media."*

Source: https://www.ftc.gov/business-guidance/resources/ftcs-endorsement-
guides-what-people-are-asking

See Figure 6.3 for appropriate marketing cues. Partnering with influencers in exchange for sponsored social media posts is a common strategy of influencer marketing used by aesthetic practices. You may engage an influencer for a one-off collaboration, or a short-term arrangement, for example, one month or longer. Determine in advance what your wish list is before reaching out or hiring an influencer management company, in terms of budget, timing, theme, etc.

Paid collaborations indicate that the influencer is posting about a brand or an entity in exchange for some consideration, either treatments, products, payments, or a combination of both. These paid collaborations are in line with traditional ads, however the personalization of the message when coming from a trusted source to their followers carries more weight than just an Instagram advert.

Thus, this form of influencer-based ads typically performs better than standard ads on Instagram, TikTok, and other platforms that are more impersonal. See Figure 6.4 for more detail on the tiers of influencers.

Determine Your Goals

Without clear goals, you won't be able to measure your success. Determine in advance what milestones you wish to achieve through partnerships with influencers and be realistic.

For long-term engagements or influencers who are represented by an agency, we always recommend executing a proper contract precisely outlining the terms of engagement to be signed by both parties, so the relationship is spelled out in detail.

A contract should have these five important terms itemized:

1. Draft a legally binding contract to engage, set expectations, define terms, #posts, where, when, content, deadlines, etc.

RELATABLE
- Influencer appeals to the target audience as a peer or is aspirational.
- Content is based on insights the audience understands and are passionate about.

AUTHENTIC
- Promotion fits into the influencer's lifestyle, image, persona.
- Influencer continues to promote your brand through multiple posts - doesn't promote competitors.

CREDIBLE
- Promoted product or service and messaging is believable.
- Influencer understands the topic & goal and can instill trust.

FIGURE 6.3 Influencer Marketing Cues

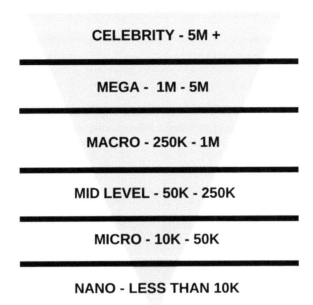

FIGURE 6.4   Influencer Tiers

2. Compensation to be itemized – payment, free treatments, products, or both.
3. Mandatory transparency – using appropriate hashtags or labels indicating that the content is paid for (to keep you both out of trouble).
4. Assign a unique code to track results (if product sales are involved).
5. Add penalties if terms are not completed satisfactorily – but be prepared not to execute these.

Of course, there can be exceptions to these policies based on your prior relationship with the influencer or a patient who may be a celebrity. You may be able to ask someone to do a Story or Reels right from your office talking about a treatment they are having.

Social Selling to Add Revenue

Social selling is trending as more key platforms are offering very advanced ways to target and sell directly to your followers. You can now sell products through Facebook Pages, Messenger, Instagram, and WhatsApp, as well as TikTok and Pinterest.

Product sales in medspas and aesthetic practices seem to have increased during and post-pandemic. This is in part due to the new, creative measures many practices adopted to sell products. During the period when procedures were prohibited in many markets, promoting products to patients was essential to keep the practice going.

Drop shipping products and curb-side pickup were great workarounds, and they seem to have stuck. In many cases, practices made sales through email marketing and text messaging, both of which help them stay in touch with patients and service their needs.

Tap into Your Community

Partnering with like-minded businesses is always a good idea. Be on the lookout for potential opportunities for leveraging local activities to promote your clinic. For example, partner with a complimentary business in your area that has a similar customer base to your own and create a collaborative deal. This can be a win-win for both businesses because it can help generate sales. Each business should leverage their own database to promote their collaboration. In this way, you are essentially sharing your resources with a non-competitive business for cross-promotion.

Another way is to team up with other professionals with whom you may share clients. For instance, an aesthetic clinic may partner with a cosmetic dentist or a popular hair salon where trendy women and men go. This strategy can help to build up both businesses in your local community and foster relationships that may lead to more referrals and collaborative efforts in the future.

Everyone likes to be a part of something that benefits their community. Try hosting a give back event during your slow season (for example, summer in some locations). Consider donating a portion of sales for a specific day or on a specific service or product to your favorite local charity. This can raise your profile within your community and spread goodwill. Your clients and staff will feel good that they are supporting a worthy cause and appreciate being connected with a business that cares about their community.

When Is it Time to Rethink Your Social Strategy?

Revisit your social channels periodically to determine whether you need to upgrade their look and feel, as well as the content you are sharing in tone, messaging, and appearance. Social trends are constantly changing, so your most important channels require some love to be effective. Let your personality come through to win hearts and minds.

Social media is the most effective way to create personal connections. Aim to meet your current and future patients where they are spending the most time, which will tend to differ from market to market.

Social media has tapped into the way we naturally build communities around topics that matter to us. Develop your community by producing relevant content in a form your audience wants to consume. This means engaging photographs, beautiful graphics and images, and more videos.

Content marketing is the path to stimulating positive conversations, building relationships and trust, and emanating empathy. Leverage your best content to nurture conversations on the most important channels that matter to your practice or medspa. This may include videos, blog posts, webinars, and more.

Keep content useful and relevant to your target audience to keep them coming back to your clinic.

7

You Are Now Entering the Metaverse

Metaverse isn't a thing a company builds. It's the next chapter of the internet overall.

Mark Zuckerberg, Founder of Meta

Why Meta?

"Meta" is "beyond" in Greek – "the next evolution of digital connection."

Meta is widely considered to be one of the most valuable companies in the world. It is among the ten largest publicly traded corporations in the US.

Since Meta is considered too big to fail, we can expect the Metaverse to continue to dominate the tech space and become more integrated into our everyday lives.

As we have seen with most big tech brands, turf wars are pretty predictable.

The Metaverse is a virtual reality where you can live in a digital world, go to work, own a house, become a businessperson, find friends, and socialize.

As of this printing, Meta owns:

- Facebook: 2.9 billion + monthly active users.
- Instagram: 2.35 billion.
- Messenger: 1.3 billion.
- WhatsApp: 2.24 billion.

Facebook demographics are:

- Largest age group – ages 25 to 34.
- Users 65+ are the smallest group on Facebook.
- 98.5% of all Facebook users are mobile users.
- 500 million + active users daily on FB Stories.

Mark Zuckerberg is known to be a little obsessed with AR and VR. The company entered this space during the pandemic and embraced it. It may have been a little too soon for the rest of us to catch on.

Remember those images of him wearing his VR goggles? Well, they are available in Meta Quest 2 and are smarter and pricier than the original. The Meta Quest 3 goggles launching in late 2023 are expected to be twice as thin and as powerful as the Quest 2. Next on the agenda, Meta plans to launch a VR headset supposedly named "Ventura," which they intend to sell "at the most attractive price point in the VR consumer market," according to endgadget.com.

Don't despair if that price is a little steep for you. Meta also launched Meta Quest gift cards that make the perfect stocking stuffer for the holidays. In fact, the Meta site is starting to look like a first cousin to Apple.

Apple launched their "Vision Pro," which is very cool. It seamlessly blends digital content with your physical space. You wear the goggles and just use your hands, eyes, and face – no screen required. It is called a "Spacial Operating System."

DOI: 10.1201/9780429356742-7

Meta for Business

If you are active on Facebook, Instagram, and WhatsApp for your business, which is essential in many markets, Meta Business Suite is where you can manage all your marketing and advertising activities on these platforms. Messenger is the other Meta platform that may be used for business. **All of these can be activated on a desktop** or mobile device, but mobile usage is by far the biggest.

The Business Suite essentially pools all your activity into one central location to help you use the Meta channels more efficiently, to achieve your marketing goals, and to connect with your followers. You can create or schedule posts, stories, and ads for your business. It is helpful to see when most of your audience is online, learn why your ad got rejected and how to troubleshoot (a common occurrence!), add someone to your account, turn on 'Professional Mode' for your profile and business and personal contacts and much more.

In essence, this Meta-only model competes with non-Meta dashboards and other tools that can pool all your social activity together, such as Sprout and Hootsuite. They offer helpful tips that are characteristically self-serving, of course. See for yourself below. It's all about the ads.

Facebook Tips Straight from the Meta Mothership

Post frequently and consistently.

- Schedule posts and stories in advance using Meta Business Suite.
- Create content in batches to save time using drafts.
- Cross-post on your Facebook and Instagram accounts to save time.
- Use the calendar view to build a regular posting schedule, fill gaps, and create engaging content using third-party templates.
- Store creative assets for your posts using Albums with Meta Business Suite. You can save them for later when you're creating content and responding to your customers' comments.

Engage with your followers.

- Prioritize your customer communications using the Updates card in your Home tab.
- Stay up to date on notifications across platforms in the Notifications tab.
- Create auto-responses to messages when answering frequently asked questions in your Inbox.
- Post content, view comments, and respond on the go with the mobile app.
- Use Inbox to respond directly to customers about the products they're asking about, or suggest others that might fit their needs.

Reach more users and followers with paid ads.

- Get to know who is engaging with your business in the Insights tab and think about how you can better define your target audience for your automated ads.
- Look at common questions and comments from followers in the Posts & Stories and Inbox tabs. These can give you clues as to what newcomers need to know about your business, which can help you understand the type of information to include in your ads to reach the target audience.
- See which of your posts drive the most engagement in the Insights tab. If you want to reach a new audience, boost it in the Posts & Stories tab.

Some practitioners and medspas may have given up on Facebook in favor of concentrating their already stretched resources on Instagram and TikTok, which are often more valuable based on their target demographic. This is an understandable strategy as no one has the resources or energy to excel on every social channel.

I still believe that Facebook is a worthwhile channel to be active on. It tends to skew older than Instagram but also shares many of the same users. It is flooded with news – some of it fake – plus a lot of ads and promotions.

The Meta army is constantly making changes to what you can and cannot post in a very arbitrary way, so it is a bit of a roller coaster ride. You really won't know how viable your content is until you post it. Content can be longer and more elaborate than on Instagram, or the same or less elaborate as you wish.

Although the majority of users access Facebook on their phones and tablets, some people will keep it open on their desktops as well. I am guilty as charged!

Caveat: Stop kidding yourself! Facebook and Instagram are ad platforms, just like Google. Social media is big business and the companies that own them are for profit business. Ads are basically a necessity to get your content seen, unless you are InstaFamous. Your content will not be seen by enough users to make a difference without boosting posts and investing in paid ads. In fact, your content may only be seen to the single digits of your followers.

Boosting a Post vs. Buying an Ad

Facebook and Instagram ads, in my experience, can be a very effective ad solution, but they require the right strategy and constant monitoring to get the most out of the spend.

A Facebook Boost Post is a paid advertisement that promotes an existing post from your business page. This amplifies the reach of your content to appear to a wider range of your target audience, beyond people who already follow your page. Boost Posts can be more limited than ad placements and audience targeting.

When choosing which posts to promote, look for the ones that get higher engagement to encourage more interactions, such as a video showcasing a popular skincare product or demonstrating a hot new trending laser treatment. You can also boost a landing page to try to get even more traffic.

By default, the platform will show your ad to users who are most likely to be interested in it. You can also segment your targeting based on interests, geography, age, previous engagement with your practice, or similarity to your most active customers.

Meta Tips

Check out Facebook Business Pages for useful intel on your account:

- See when most of your audience is online.
- Find out why your ad got rejected and how to troubleshoot.
- How to add someone to your account.
- Learn how to turn on Professional Mode for your profile for your business and personal contacts.

Geo-Targeting

Geo-targeting allows you to target potential customers in a specific area based on country, region, or city. Facebook can be a good platform for advertising.

Meta has made it simpler to target the people you want to get in front of by allowing businesses to display their ads exactly where those audiences are.

Six Tips for Getting Results from Facebook

1. Create a business page for your practice or medspa. Keep personal pages separate from your business pages on all channels to avoid confusion and cross-over from users.

2. Target the audience you want to reach with video and static ads and boosted posts.

3. Try Facebook Stories, which are like Instagram Stories, but not as overused.

4. Facebook Live can be used for hosting virtual events and demonstrations, but Instagram Live is a better option. Neither of these features are nearly as popular as they were pre-TikTok.

5. Create a steady stream of videos and compelling images to get traction. Videos that do best are native to Facebook, as opposed to pulling videos from an external source. On all channels, video rules!

6. Unlike many platforms, negative comments can be deleted, blocked, hidden, and flagged to Facebook. However, don't expect a response from Meta any time in the next century...

#InstaFamous

Instagram is still killing it as a tool for growing aesthetic practices and medspas.

In many markets, including the US, the UK, and Canada, for example, Instagram is rated as either the most valuable platform for aesthetic practices, or next after TikTok, depending on whom you ask and what kind of practice or medspa they have.

It differs from Facebook as it is an app and has site-specific limitations in terms of scheduling content, ads, promotions, and content formats. However, the two platforms are connected, which makes it easier to share and repurpose content.

The largest group of users on Instagram are under 30 and are not likely to spend much time on Facebook. Depending on location, they have also flocked to TikTok as their channel of choice in markets where it is popular. This powerful audience also watches a lot of YouTube videos.

Considered the most valuable platform for aesthetic surgery and dermatology practices in many markets, TikTok may exceed Instagram in some markets. Instagram offers key features that are most relevant to primary and secondary target demographics in the aesthetic market.

Five Things to Know About Instagram Users

1. Women use it more than men.

2. It is the most popular channel among younger audiences (18 to 34) but in some markets TikTok may be the front runner

3. Reels have the highest reach – more than Feed and Stories.

4. Following and researching brands is the second most popular activity.

5. Users prefer Stories with a mix of photos, videos, text, quizzes, polls, etc.

Source: https://sproutsocial.com/insights/instagram-stats/

If you are not active on Instagram in many markets, your practice may not be visible to the patients you want to attract.

Users can find a plethora of content devoted to topics that dovetail with what aesthetic clinics and medical spas specialize in.

- Beauty.
- Skincare.
- Spa treatments.
- Lasers.
- Injectables.
- Hair care.
- Fitness trends.
- Cosmetic surgery (not only BBL and breast implants).

Designing a Cohesive Channel

More than most other platforms, Instagrammers have high standards for beautiful photos, engaging content, and welcome a cohesive-looking channel.

Tips for a Beautiful IG

- Define your audience.
- Use a color scheme and brand colors.
- Image content.
- Schedule posting and be consistent.
- TOV (tone of voice).
- Get your font right.
- Tell your story.
- Match your feed to your bio.
- Mix it up. Use reels in your grid. Use videos, infographics, and memes. Follow the trends that matter to your target audience.

Caveat: Posting long paragraphs of text may backfire as users view Instagram almost exclusively on their phones. Images speak louder than text. Try to avoid "Scroll Down" as it may be too much work for many users to bother so they will never see it.

Optimizing Your Profile

Although the character count for descriptions on Instagram is limited, make the most of every other option to broaden your visibility.

Use the most important words in the description: who you are, what you do, and how to find you – website, email, text, etc.

Let followers know that you offer virtual consults and any other details that can make your practice stand out.

Add Your "Link in Bio" to drive traffic from Instagram. If you are having a special offer or want to drive visitors somewhere more specific rather than just your URL. You can change the Link in Bio any time. This is a very valuable too so take full advantage of it.

INSTAGRAM BIO LINK TOOLS

Instagram Bio Link is a landing page where you can consolidate all your important links, including photos, videos, articles, endorsements, honors, etc.

Linktree: Most popular tool for adding links in your bio.
Shor.by: Used to create a micro landing page with multiple links to your content and social profiles or add blocks like buttons or cards, schedule posts, and create a dynamic feed to automatically post your latest content.
Pally: A scheduling program that also features a customized Instagram Bio Link Tool.

Six Ways to Take Advantage of Highlights

Instagram highlights are the thematic collections of your stories that live at the bottom of your profile. Stories can be saved to your profile by adding them to Highlights, or they will disappear in 24 hours.

1. Personalize your highlights with your branding to stand out and make them your own. Keep in mind that these are going to be viewed on a tiny phone so make sure they are legible.
2. Label your highlights to share unique information and details, such as Clinic News, Our Team, Before-and-After photos, Individual members, New treatments, etc.
3. Change your covers for special promotions, seasonal treatments, relevant holidays, clinic milestones.
4. Proudly promotes your accolades: studies you have done, media mentions, speaking engagements, meetings attended, and more.
5. Pull previously posted content to add to the appropriate highlights or add a story post to the highlight while posting.
6. Use highlights for promoting newsworthy topics: announcements, events, new products or services, or anything else you want your followers to know about you as a practitioner and your practice or medspa.

Cool Instagram Features

- The most powerful ways to gain Instagram popularity are Reels, Stories, and Feed, in descending order.
- Video performs very well on Instagram.
- IG users tend to have pretty high standards for images and videos. So, if it doesn't look great on a phone, don't post it, at least on that channel.
- Your Feed should look cohesive to represent your image and brand in the best possible way.
- You can add posts with multiple pages, a cover photo for your videos, and use line breaks in your captions and bio.
- You may choose to use a branded color scheme, the same filter for all images, as well as branded formats for patient photos, videos, and other types of posts to distinguish your Feed from everything else.
- Check out the most popular hacks to help create a unique style and stand out from the crowd.

Designing a Cohesive Feed

- Post directly to your Feed and/or to Stories.
- In your Feed, posts can be landscape, square, portrait, or a mix of both.
- Video is a critical success factor on Instagram and gets better engagement than static posts.
- Use captions to provide useful information for your followers – how-to instructions, detailed explanations of treatments, how to apply skincare products, and information about images posted.
- The best times to post are when your target audiences are most active on the platform; there is no universal day or time, and every market is different.

Tips to Ace Your Instagram Channel

Instagram only allows a clickable link in your bio to direct visitors to your website or anywhere else, but it can be changed any time to direct viewers to another URL.

You can also add a launchpad link which allows you to share multiple links on social.

Add your location to be found locally.

Static posts tend to get less engagement because they can be dull; videos are far more effective in Feed and Stories

Always add a call-to-action (CTA): What do you want the viewer to do after seeing your post? Call, text, share, etc.

A DOZEN TOOLS YOU CAN USE

Make your Instagram look like a pro did it

1. *Adobe Light Room lightroom.adobe.com*
2. *Snapseed https://snapseed.online/*
3. *Picsart picsart.com*
4. *Visco visco.co*
5. *Pixler pixlr.com*
6. *Polarr polarr.com*
7. *Afterlight afterlight.co*
8. *TouchRetouch Object Removal*
9. *Instasize instasize.com*
10. *Musecam musecam.co*
11. *CreatorKit https://creatorkit.com/*
12. *Cutout.Pro https://www.cutout.pro/*

AI apps for photos are a great way to give your photos personalized retouches and to hide flaws using modern AI features.

Five AI Photo Apps to Try

1. Filmora.
2. Lensa AI.
3. Remini – AI Photo Enhancer.
4. PhotoDirector.
5. Fotor AI Image Editor.

Five Al Background Generators

1. PhotoRoom – photoroom.com/
2. Fotor – fotor.com
3. Hotpot – https://hotpot.ai/
4. CreatorKit – https://creatorkit.com/
5. Appy Pie Design – appypie.com

Engaging on Instagram

Aesthetic patients will often reach out to doctors, nurses, aestheticians, and clinic staff through direct messages (DMs). These should be monitored 24/7 and responded to in real-time, if possible.

- Follow what your patients are promoting.
- Communicate through comments and DMs.
- Get notifications when users you follow post new content.
  - Visit the profile page of the account you want to get notifications for.
  - Tap the three dots in the upper right corner of the screen.
  - Select 'Turn on Post Notifications'.
- Share posts from friends or patients (with consent) in your feed on Stories.
  - Click on the paper airplane icon below the post.
  - Tap Add post to your story.
  - The post will appear as a sticker with a custom background.
- Add a story you are mentioned in by another user to your own story.

Instagram Stories

To put the importance of Stories in perspective, these are viewed by over 500 million users daily. Creating interactive stories, asking your audience questions, or adding quizzes and polls can all boost your engagement.

At the time of this printing, Stories have a lifespan of 24 hours and videos can run for up to 15 seconds. However, you can split a longer video into 15-second segments, if desired. Stories can get great engagement and help to generate interest in your Feed to more users.

Eight Tips for Amazing Stories

1. Share multiple photos and videos that appear together in a slideshow format or Reel.
2. Lives last for 24 hours in your Feed, profile, and direct – add it as a Highlight to keep it forever.
3. Add to your Stories and repurpose snippets to other channels. Share photos and videos from your Story to Feed.
4. Cross-promote content from TikTok or Facebook on your Instagram channel.
5. Add fonts, coloring tools, boomerangs, and stickers.
6. The best tone tends to be upbeat and creative.
7. Once you reach 10,000 followers, add a swipe-up link to your website to boost traffic.
8. Repurpose snippets of photos, text and videos from other channels to your stories, and vice versa.

Instagram Live

Lives can be a good way to engage followers and encourage them to tag their friends for more engagement. Enticing them with a gift card raffle can help spark more attendees.

There is little to no preparation, and you can just relax and talk about a topic that you and your followers are interested in. These require some promotion to get good attendance. Since they are short – 30 to 45 minutes typically – guests may stick around if they are interested in the topic and the discussion is lively, entertaining, or informative. Offer an incentive to 'invite a friend' too.

Instagram Live stream time is limited to one hour so you need to log off before the 60-minute mark. Be sure to save your Live to your camera roll so you can add it to IGTV. Otherwise, your Live will only last for 24 hours. Once you get the hang of setting it up, you are good to go. It may take a while to build traction with these events but if you can get it going, it may open some doors.

Be Prepared with Talking Points

- If you're showing off a product, treatment, or specific topic, have some relevant facts or stats to share that viewers will be interested in.
- If you're interviewing someone, jot down a couple questions ahead of time so you don't blank while recording. Let the audience know that they can ask questions in real-time during the Live.
- Remind followers of who you are and who your guest is throughout the video in case new users come on and miss your introduction.
- If you're live streaming an event or presentation, an explanation helps to engage the audience throughout.
- Type a title for your live video in the comments section at the bottom of the screen.
- Once you share a comment, you can tap to pin it to the screen.

Fifteen Tips for Hosting a Virtual Event on Instagram Live

1. Choose a trending theme to keep it interesting.
2. Promote it in advance – but not too far in advance so users forget.
3. Create a countdown on IG Stories.
4. Schedule the live stream in advance and add it to a post.
5. Use a targeted Instagram promotion to attract a local audience.
6. Incorporate Q&A into the interview format.
7. Add question stickers in Stories before the Live so you can gather questions to answer during the live call.
8. Offer giveaways, samples, virtual consults, and special pricing to select attendees.
9. Incorporate demonstrations of products and treatments as well as virtual tours of your clinic.
10. Encourage audience questions to increase engagement.
11. Use "practice mode" if you want to test it in advance to get the tech down.
12. Use the "add a friend" feature to create a more engaging experience and to extend the reach of your live stream.
13. Share your video in your Story and add to Feed. Make sure you add the video on your camera roll so you can share it on other platforms, send it, or replay yourself.
14. Reiterate your purpose and end your live stream with some call-to-action that ties back to your goals and objectives.
15. Choose the winner or winners of the event at the end and announce the date and time for the next event.

Mastering Reels

Reels is basically Meta's way of offering a TikTok-like feature to users and steering some of the app's traction to stick with Instagram.

Try to maximize your Reels reach by aligning with these three strategies:

1. Determine which Reels to show on the best day and time.
2. Look at your history, activity, and process information within Reels.
3. Avoid promoting low-resolution content which will not perform well.

Reels can attract a lot of viewers and increase the number of visits to your profile, even if they don't interact with your posts. The content of your Reel should be unique, include helpful information that adds value, and make the audience feel connected to your brand.

The more Reels a viewer watches – ideally all the way through – the more sign of interest Instagram can use to determine what they want to see. Likes, frequency, and quality of comments may also play a role.

If you create your own Reels like those you watch that have good traction, you can see more of that type of content as well. Instagram tracks what you engage with by showing you more content like what you have already watched based on their AI system. Thus, users who engage with videos about injectable treatments are likely see more Reels about fillers and toxins. Meta's video identification algorithms are always changing, so check back frequently to read about any updates.

While sharing clips from TikTok may seem like an obvious play, it can work against you. Instagram's AI can detect when videos are shared by competitors and may limit their reach. However, the tone of content for both short-form video platforms set to music is very similar and tends to be light, upbeat, and entertaining.

You can repurpose content to share on both channels by making some tweaks. For example, choose different music or use a 30-second clip of a 60-second video, etc. Use your creativity to make it work. Ideally it is worthwhile to be active on both of these very important channels.

Caveat: Keep in mind that each of these platforms work differently and has its own ethos. Instagram is not YouTube, for example, and their users log on for different reasons. Don't try to apply the same strategy to every channel you are active on because it may backfire on you.

Consistently creating quality, engaging content can be a challenge for busy practitioners. This is a task that may be best delegated to staff members or outsourced to an external team if it cannot be handled internally as needed. To learn what may work best, follow high-profile channels on Instagram, TikTok, and Snapchat to get ideas and jumpstart better engagement.

There are constant updates and changes coming from all social platforms, which makes it hard to stay on top of everything. Instagram and TikTok are highly competitive, so when one of these platforms changes the rules or adds another feature that takes off, the other is likely to follow. For example, Instagram Reels went from 15 seconds to 30 seconds. TikTok enables the upload of longer clips of up to 3 minutes and YouTube Shorts can be up to 60 minutes. Instagram expanded the maximum time for Reels to 60 seconds.

Ten Tips for Mastering Reels

1. Reels is a similar format to TikTok with short, fun, lively videos set to music.
2. Choose music from IG's music library or create your own.
3. Reels allows up to 60 seconds but this is subject to change.
4. A big advantage is that it lives on the Instagram platform for ease of use.
5. You can be active on both Reels and TikTok. In fact, I would recommend that.
6. When you share your Reel, it will live on a separate Reels tab on your profile where users can find it.
7. If you share your Reel to your Feed, it will appear on your main profile grid – but you have the option to remove it.
8. If you share a Reels to a Story, it will disappear in 24 hours.
9. Reels are a good way to highlight a new treatment or product in your clinic.
10. It can help to get the whole clinic team involved in creating enough content to keep your Reels active.

Messenger

Key Feature: Chat Themes at the End-to-end Encryption

Messenger is pretty much what its name implies, a platform connecting people through texting, videos, and calls. Facebook, as it was called then, picked up this app in 2010.

Fairly recently, Meta started incorporating "chat themes at the end-to-end encryption" with plans to roll it out to more countries. This is a big step up for business users and will make it easier to converse with patients and clients because of the privacy upgrade.

Users can customize their responses with emojis and selfie stickers, plus AR features. It also allows the ability to use group chats to communicate with peers, friends, and co-workers.

If you are an Apple (IOS) user, you can use the face or fingerprint ID on your phone to unlock Messenger and keep all your chats private.

Don't get too excited yet. The sudden attention Meta is giving to Messenger indicates one important trend: they are looking for ways to monetize the channel for business users.

It was bound to happen sooner or later.

WhatsApp

Key Feature: End-to-End Encryption

I love WhatsApp with one annoying exception: I constantly get unsolicited sales pitches for lasers from Asian companies, and even when I block and delete them, they find their way back into my feed.

WhatsApp has a lot of cool features that work for business and personal use. For those of us who travel abroad, it's a great way to stay in touch with friends, staff, and colleagues, or even Uber drivers and concierges when needed.

You can use the platform online or on your desktop to chat, even when your phone is off (or you misplaced it). Meta launched a broadcast-based messaging feature called "Channels" on WhatsApp most likely to try to jumpstart more opportunities for conversations and encourage more business users to monetize the app.

What's Trending on Meta

It takes a small army to keep up with the trends on every platform you choose to be active on. In fact, what may have been trending when I penned this chapter, can potentially be obsolete by the time you read it.

While the notion of the Metaverse may still be confusing to many of us, it seems like it is here to stay. Zuckerberg appears to be committed to making this his baby and seeing it through.

5 Trends to Follow in the Metaverse

- VR head gear to attract more users
- AR gadgets and AR enabled devices
- Virtual storefronts, offices and meeting rooms
- Avatars and assistants powered by AI
- Consumers creating their own avatars (Figure 7.1).

Virtual Reality (VR)

VR creates a totally artificial environment so users can experience a real-world environment. It generates related information that is overlaid on top of it. VR uses headsets that fit over your head and simulate visual and audio information.

For example, the Meta Quest Pro is based on VR.

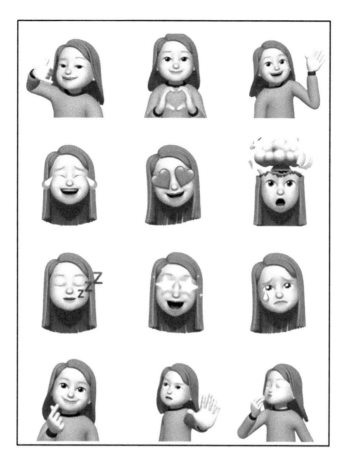

FIGURE 7.1 Consumers experimenting with creating avatars.

AR VS. VR

Augmented Reality (AR) completely immerses users in a virtual environment. That augmented reality uses the existing real-world environment and puts virtual information on top of it. It places the user in a sort of mixed reality with a new, simulated environment.

Virtual Reality (VR) is a virtual environment created with software that is presented to users in a way that lets their brains suspend belief long enough to accept a virtual world as a real environment. Virtual reality is primarily experienced through a headset with sight and sound.

Augmented Reality (AR)

Augmented reality uses the existing real-world environment and puts virtual information on top of it. AR can use devices like phones, glasses, and projections. It also works with HUDs in cars. These are projectors embedded in the dashboard that send a transparent image onto the windscreen by bouncing off a series of mirrors before being magnified so it is legible to drivers.

Source: https://www.techtarget.com

Apple's Vision Pro, referred to as 'Apple's First Spatial Operating System' which is their first augmented reality (AR) headset, is not even referred to as AR or VR. It hit the market in February, 2024 and is pretty amazing.

I signed up to be notified when it will be available, which is expected to be 2024 at a hefty price tag. Check it out because it's pretty amazing, but kind of terrifying at the same time.

Virtual Stores

Virtual shopping is an e-commerce service for customers to make purchases in a virtual environment – as if they were in an actual store. AR and VR technologies as well as 3D models may be used to create these Virtual Reality stores. For example, consider how your business may benefit from what Meta offers because it is still the biggest and most profitable platform to date. Meta is committed to this concept as a long-term money-maker.

Get to Know Super Apps

Super apps combine various features. This may include messaging, video, entertainment, commerce, or payment.

This offers users more immersive experiences and the benefits of addressing multiple needs in a single platform.

- TikTok has been adding multiple features that directly copy other social media apps like carousels, stories, and longer videos, and is making moves into the non-digital world.
- Meta has changed reimagined WhatsApp to go beyond just one-on-one messaging by adding community tools and payment features in selected regions.
- These features can be used to give your followers a more convenient, all-in-one experience on your social platforms.

Social Media for Customer Service

More businesses are incorporating a customer service element in their social media strategies. This means using social media as a direct line of communication with customers, to quickly address questions, complaints, and requests. It is also important to proactively respond to customers who mention your brand – both positively and negatively.

Since more potential clients are active on these channels, offering support via the platforms they are on is a good way to help to enhance customer service.

Platforms like Facebook offer features such as a common inbox, automated responses, and chatbots to simplify customer service management and improve response times, which can help you grow your brand.

Public responses may show that you care about your clients and patients, which can build trust and transparency. Ignoring inquiries or complaints on an open forum can have a negative impact on your online reputation. Viewers may assume that your brand is not interested in engaging and may not reach out.

Four Ways to Weave Customer Service into Your Social Strategy

1. Open your social media DMs for visitors to submit questions and complaints. Be sure that someone is monitoring any comments that may arise to respond as close to real-time as possible.
2. Follow the lead of some hotel brands and airlines and set up separate, dedicated channels for customer support. If you choose to do this, they need to be managed 24 hours and 7 days per week.
3. If you offer customer support in a public forum (X (formerly Twitter) for example), it may be best to take the conversation offline so it can be dealt with in private.
4. If you have engaged an external social media team, keep them up to speed on your practice's customer service methods for consistency.

Eight Hot Social Trends to Add to Your Marketing Plan

1. Social commerce (Meta, TikTok).
2. Short-form videos (TikTok, YouTube Shorts).
3. Long-form videos (YouTube, websites, blogs).
4. Augmented reality (AR).
5. Virtual reality (VR).
6. Micro-influencers (Instagram, TikTok, YouTube).
7. Paid creators (Instagram, TikTok, YouTube).
8. Omnichannel marketing (all channels, etc.).

Super Helpful Business Tips for Ten Key Channels

These are updated frequently to keep you up to speed on the best and brightest features to tap into.

Facebook: https://www.facebook.com/business/tools/meta-business-suite

Instagram: https://business.instagram.com/

LinkedIn: https://business.linkedin.com/marketing-solutions/linkedin-pages

Pinterest: https://business.pinterest.com/

Snapchat: https://forbusiness.snapchat.com/en-US

TikTok: https://business.tiktok.com/

Twitter: https://business.twitter.com/

WeChat: https://www.wechat.com/

WhatsApp: https://business.whatsapp.com/

YouTube: https://www.youtube.com/'

NOTE: Check into these helpful business tips regularly; social media channels changes constantly and there is always more to learn.

Figure 7.2 shows four ways to maintain your online presence.

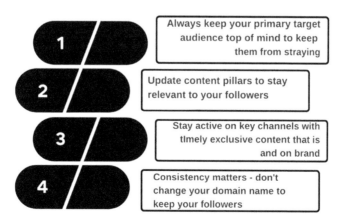

4 Key Ways to Maintain Your Online Presence

1. Always keep your primary target audience top of mind to keep them from straying
2. Update content pillars to stay relevant to your followers
3. Stay active on key channels with tImely exclusive content that is and on brand
4. Consistency matters - don't change your domain name to keep your followers

FIGURE 7.2 Four ways to maintain your online presence.

Managing Complaints and Negative Reviews

In a competitive marketplace and considering the many platforms consumers can use to voice their opinions online, managing consumer complaints is a critical success factor.

Think of it this way. There is an opportunity to learn from clients who complain. They may be pointing out something you are unaware of. The worst thing you can do is ignore complaints or get defensive. It is possible to turn it around to make the complaining client become an advocate, but this may take some patience and a lot of eating crow.

It is important to always take negative feedback seriously rather than let it fester and boil. In aesthetics, handling client complaints or concerns needs to be a ten out of ten. Of course, that may not be feasible 100% of the time but strive to get as close as you can.

One unflattering negative review can bring your rating down, which can hurt you in the public eye. In my opinion, any review that scores less than four out of five stars is a liability. Make sure your patients understand that. While they may think that a 4 or 4.5 is just fine, 5 star reviews are what you need to be shooting for.

It is a good idea to let patients and clients know what sites are the most important for your business. For example, if your Google or Facebook reviews are hurting, try to steer patients to post on these platforms first.

> *To prove my point, we looked at several review sites to see what kind of negative reviews aesthetic patients were posting...*
> > *Here are some random patient complaints found on review sites*
> > *Don't be surprised if some of these sound eerily familiar...*
>
> - *They weren't hearing me when I explained what I wanted.*
> - *The staff didn't make me feel welcome and rushed me.*
> - *They overcharged me for my treatment and ignored me when I said something.*
> - *The results were too aggressive. I didn't even look like myself and the bruising took a week to go down.*
> - *I didn't see any difference from the injections and it wasn't worth the money. I wouldn't go back.*
> - *I told the nurse that I didn't want my boyfriend to know I had anything done and I had a big bruise under my eye when I left.*
> - *The laser treatment was ok but they tried to sell me on a series of treatment but I wasn't having it. I wouldn't go back there.*
> - *Terrible experience! They rushed me out of the room for another patient.*
> - *DO NOT go to this clinic. They overcharge for treatments and are very pushy to get me to sign up for more.*

In my experience, it is less common for consumer complaints to be just about the treatment or outcome. It is more likely to be about their experience. Another common topic is fees or payments.

Isn't it better to know when you didn't do a great job for one reason or another than to live in ignorance and let it happen again? Turning an unhappy client into a loyal customer is possible, but you must be aware of their complaints so you can address them head-on.

This is why automated follow-up texts or email questionnaires, like airlines and hotels use, are helpful to flag unhappy clients. Ideally, someone in the practice should be assigned to manage this process, and all staff should be trained in how best to handle patients who are unhappy. There is a short window to turn angry patients around, so the whole staff should be mindful of this.

Social Listening

Social listening is a vital exercise for every business and brand.

In short, if you don't listen to what your audience wants and needs, you may be missing the opportunity to connect to help or influence them. It is a common mistake for practices to assume they know exactly what their patients or clients want without ever asking them directly. Thus, you may be making tactical moves without the benefit of getting hard evidence to guide you instead of strategic decisions.

It is important to learn what your audience is saying about you to stay on top of it. You may be living in ignorance and miss out on the opportunity to improve your public persona.

Yet, social listening can be a double-edged sword. Try not to approach this useful exercise by being defensive. Keep an open mind so you can obtain valuable intel on what may need improvement.

If you read negative comments from someone you believe is a real patient, do not respond in a public forum as that would be considered a privacy violation. It is always best to move the discussion offline if possible. If you can identify the complaining patient, you could try to invite them back to your practice and address their dissatisfaction in person.

Caveat: *As a licensed medical professional, it is unwise (I am being kind here) to post or respond to anything that acknowledges a doctor-patient relationship in an open forum. Always try to take the conversation offline!*

Monitoring Your Online Reputation – Webtools

- The best practice is that whoever did the treatment (doctor, nurse, etc.) should ask happy patients personally if they are willing to write a review and share their experience with others online.

- Make it as easy as possible for patients to write a review. Try QR codes they can scan, a link you send them as a text message that they can click and start writing, or an email. Make sure it gets to them as soon as possible.

- Some systems can be connected with your practice management software to automate review requests. Birdeye and Solution Reach (in the US) and others will send requests for reviews on your behalf to patients who visit the practice.

- GoogleMyBusiness is very visible in search results. If more patients write reviews about your clinic there, it will elevate your listing when potential patients are looking for a provider in your area. Google prefers seeing recent reviews that contain the name of the treatment the patient had. Note that for a patient to post a review on Google, they need to sign into (or open) a Google account. Some patients are concerned about their privacy and may be reluctant to use an account with their real full name.

- For other review sites that may be popular in your market (Yelp, TrustPilot, Facebook, etc.), direct patients to these platforms to write about their experience. Patients can upload photos and videos to some of these websites, and the system's algorithm may choose to show your listing more often when you accumulate rich, detailed reviews.

- Each review platform has content guidelines and terms of use. If you find that a negative review does not match these guidelines and would like it modified or removed, try to get in touch with their content team and explain your reasoning. Include quotes from their policy and an explanation for why certain sentences may not adhere to their guidelines. For example, Yelp doesn't want to see the same review on another site and may remove it or contact the author if the content is not unique.

Source: https://webtoolsgroup.com/

8

Multimedia Communication in Action

Listen more than you talk. Nobody learned anything by hearing themselves speak.

Richard Branson, Founder of Virgin Group

A Multimedia Strategy

Staying on top of the trends in marketing for your practice or medspa takes a village, but it's worth the effort.

By implementing a multimedia strategy, you can leverage a select mix of targeted complementary channels. One of the profound benefits of this concept is that the percentage of the total target audience increases.

The forms of communication you choose to be active with should be the ones that resonate with your current clients and patients, as well as your key target audience.

This increases the percentage of the total target audience that a programmatic campaign reaches. A multichannel strategy is becoming increasingly crucial in today's programmatic landscape because consumers are active across various channels and devices (Figure 8.1).

Multi-Sensory Social Media

Multi-sensory social media refers to utilizing various formats including audio, video, text, and images to create a more engaging experience for users. Instagram now features an option to add music to still images. Editing content to include audio, polls, music, captions, and other formats taps into the concept of multi-sensory social media.

Four Ways to Create Multi-Sensory Social Posts

- **Text**: Text is still a primary way of creating and sharing information, and it can also be used to augment other forms of communication, such as descriptions on photos.
- **Photos**: Text and images can be combined in a single form. Many apps and software programs make it easy to create graphics that combine a strong visual element.
- **Audio**: Sound files can be compressed to reduce the file size without sacrificing sound quality. Compressed files are easier to store and stream faster when shared.
- **Video:** Video typically combines images and sound for a compelling multimedia experience. Videos can include text as well, in the form of captions or as text in an image.

DOI: 10.1201/9780429356742-8

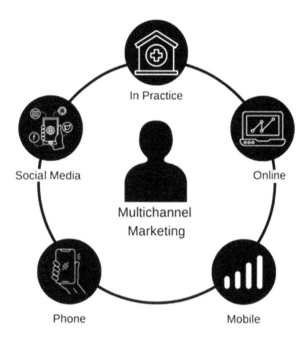

FIGURE 8.1   Multichannel marketing

Content Driven by Data

For most small to mid-size businesses, the following communication vehicles are the most practical and affordable to take advantage of. They also cast the widest net. I included VR and AR because these important developments are emerging as the next frontier in communications.

Communications in Practice

1. Text
2. Images
3. Video
4. Audio (podcast, radio)
5. Virtual reality (VR)
6. Augmented reality (AR)

Go Straight to Video

Think video first, or at the very least, second.

If you are not all-in with video content across all your social channels, as well as your practice website, you are missing out on a critical success factor for your marketing plan.

If you have the bandwidth, aim to have a presence on the most popular platforms for short-form videos because that is what is trending globally. These include Instagram (Reels), TikTok, and YouTube (Shorts). Create your own brand channel and/or work directly with the right local or regional influencer to whom your target audience relates.

Not surprisingly, other platforms were eager to make video their default option too. Everyone copies everything in the highly competitive landscape of digital marketing.

Explaining Explainer Videos

The term "explainer video" is like a techie way to say "how to's."

These are typically short-form videos created to "explain" a product, treatment, or service to patients and clients. It is a very powerful yet simple strategy to engage clients and entice them to want to try what you are featuring.

I like to suggest that you choose a format to use for a series of these simple videos so they can be ownable. These can be about what something is, how to do it, what are the benefits, when to take action, and any other themes that dovetail well into practices and medspa agendas.

An explainer video is simply a short film that communicates how something works in a simple and straightforward way. They are typically used as marketing videos to demonstrate the benefits of a product or service and to boost sales or sign-ups. They can also be used to share outcomes, demonstrate a consultation, or document the patient experience.

Consider these videos to be a modern visual alternative to the paper brochures many practices still have at the front desk or in their treatment rooms. Some patients may flip through these while they are waiting, but mostly they tend to leave in the restroom or toss them into the nearest trashcan on their way out the door.

Remember: Aim to ditch paper materials in your practice. This will upgrade and modernize your business, and you may save a few trees in the process. GenZ and millenials will notice that you care about the environment.

When we work with practices, we eliminate all paper materials possible, except toilet paper and paper towels. We don't even like to see old-school glossy bifold or trifold brochures left by sales reps to promote their products anymore.

Paper is just not the way you want to go in 2024!

Five Simple Video Themes to Try:

1. **Demonstrate how to do something**: Show how to use a product properly, aftercare from a laser treatment, post-procedure skincare application, what to do before and after an injectable treatment, healthy eating tips, and the list goes on.
2. **Showcase your best outcomes**: Everyone loves to show beautiful results, and patients are keen to see your work. Mix up the photos you select to show different ages and skin tones so patients will know that your patients are diverse.
3. **In their own words**: Share an interview with one of your patients speaking about their experience in your practice and how they feel about their treatment.
4. **Tape a mock consultation**: Give prospective patients a sneak peek at how you conduct a consultation. Evaluate patients so they know what to expect and feel comfortable scheduling an appointment.
5. **Film a live treatment in your practice**: Walk the viewer through the process of before-and-after a treatment and explain the steps through the experience.

How to use videos is shown in Figure 8.2.

Trend Alert: Short-form Videos

Short-form videos are hot and are predicted to continue to exceed in popularity. These days, most humans have a limited tolerance for anything that is longer than a few seconds, so take that on board.

By short I mean really short, as in videos of 5 to 30 seconds maximum, which speaks to our increasingly limited attention spans. These mini-videos or snippets can grab viewers' attention instantly and keep them engaged with your channel.

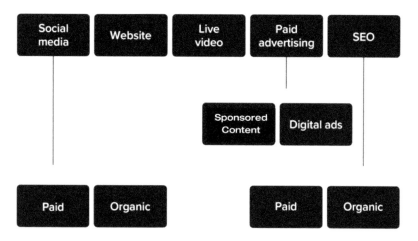

FIGURE 8.2   How to use video

Among the best channels to experiment with are TikTok, YouTube Shorts, and Instagram Reels and Stories. Short videos are also popular on LinkedIn and Facebook.

Pinterest is another site to check out if you are active on this social platform. I am disappointed that this site seems to be forgotten. I consider it to be very underused and you may find that you can acquire follower who can be diverted to your main channels in the process.

Five Simple Short Form Video Ideas to Try

1. Demos of new or combination treatments.
2. How-to's for skincare application and usage.
3. "Behind the scenes" snippets of your practice at work.
4. Teasers to introduce a new injectable or laser treatment.
5. Patient reviews and testimonials.

You may also see these trending in paid media to increase clicks to your website and stimulate more leads.

Using Video Across All Channels

Video plays a pivotal role as part of a comprehensive marketing plan. It has emerged as a key strategy on every platform, and the sky is the limit as to how you may use them to your advantage. In fact, not using video is a mistake that will cost you in terms of engagement and attracting more fans and followers.

Great video content has become the preferred way of informing and connecting with your audience. Never underestimate the power of a brilliant video campaign to inform and entertain audiences across all age groups and users.

Some common ways to use videos include explainer videos, which teach the viewer how to do something, social media content, and presentations including slide decks and webinars. It can be repurposed for just about everywhere you use written content such as for your blog, website, all social media channels, text messaging, etc.

If you are not comfortable with taking videos with your phone, there are numerous tools and apps that can make the process easier and more effective. Good quality video with the right lighting makes a big difference.

The versatility of video is limited only by your bandwidth. Use short-form videos across every channel, on your blog and website, on the monitors in your waiting room and patient areas, and anywhere else that is patient-facing.

Long-Form Video

Video is where it's at across demographics and age groups.

It is considered the preferred way to get information across, as well as for entertainment. The shorter the better for younger demographics. However, more mature audiences also appreciate educational videos that tell a story or teach them something useful.

Long-form video is a vital component of a modern website so patients can get to know your practice before they ever make an appointment. Keep them short and simple, such as 60 second, for your website and blogs.

On YouTube, you can stretch it out much longer. Test out several lengths to determine what your primary audience likes best.

15- to 30-second videos tend to be the sweet spot for most demographics. Try extending content to 60 seconds and up for a more mature audience who may prefer more detailed interesting content to spend their time on.

Any length of video may work depending on the subject, the quality of the footage, and your platform of choice. Versatility is what makes A-list video content a smart investment for your marketing plan. Never underestimate the power of a brilliant video campaign to inform and entertain audiences across age groups.

DIVERSIFY YOUR STORYTELLING

1. *Create videos to be viewed on mobile devices, tablets, phones, and Apple watches for users on the move.*
2. *Repurpose your videos for all social channels, websites, and blogs.*
3. *Long-form videos can be used on your practice's website so patients can feel like they know your practice.*
4. *Short-form videos tend to get more views and can be repurposed for all channels. Change out the captions, first frame, and title as needed.*
5. *Live video content (TikTok, YouTube, IG Reels) encourages more engagement. Add text to frames for viewers who keep the sound off in public.*
6. *Play videos on monitors (sound off) in waiting rooms and treatment rooms for patient education.*

YouTube, the Original All-Video Platform

Owned by Google, YouTube was into all video a few decades before TikTok came along.

YouTube is a free to use video-sharing service where users can watch, like, share, comment, and upload their own videos. Young tweens and teens use it to watch music videos, TV shows, how to guides, recipes, hair and makeup vloggers, and YouTube's version of influencers.

To grow a successful YouTube channel, owners must pay close attention to their audience, analytics, and SEO which are crucial to boosting their ranking. The most well-ranking YouTube channels tend to stick to a theme that may range from travel, tutorials, beauty, or their daily lives. Viewers like to engage with interesting, unique content that tends to be personal.

The channel is all about connecting, sharing, and collaborating with other users. To be successful, users need to build their network through constant video posts, so it takes a lot of work to get there.

YouTube shorts are a relatively new feature that help users to connect with more viewers. Shorts were introduced to mimic Instagram Reels and TikTok videos. YouTube shorts are traditionally shot in a vertical orientation and are 60 seconds or less to be easily viewed on a smartphone.

How to Use Memes and GIFs

Memes: Pronounced "meem," this typically features text over an existing image, and the key message can highlight something that is humorous or relatable about the image.

Memes can be used to offer commentary on a topic in a visual and usually humorous way. You can get your point across with an amusing image and a short caption that is typically up to 25 characters.

GIFs: GIF, pronounced with a hard G, is short for "graphics interchange format file." In its simplest form, a GIF is an image file that can be used to create animated images.

Ten GIF Tips

1. Your GIF should serve a purpose, such as guiding viewers to your call-to-action (CTA).
2. Use the first frame to clearly communicate your key message.
3. Show a series of steps in a process.
4. Show cause and effect.
5. Showcase patient photos.
6. Illustrate comparisons.
7. Share mini demos.
8. Social media teasers.
9. Quick tips (Skincare, products, etc).
10. Add "Fast Facts."

Source: https://forgeandsmith.com/blog/top-10-tips-to-pick-the-perfect
-gif/#2_Know_your_pop_culture

Dissecting Media Formats

Print Media

Print media may be a mainstay at some news organizations, but readership has been steadily declining, especially among younger generations. Many print publications have folded full stop, or have ceased print versions in favor of subscription-based digital content.

Depending on your market, the UK being one of them, print can be used to share information with an older demographic. It is also the most expensive model for creating marketing content for your business. Some practices and medspas may do a quarterly or semi-annual magazine to reach an older population in the community and as something to read in the waiting room. The downsides are production costs, time spent producing the content, and postage if you plan to mail it out. The upside is that you can repurpose the content for a digital version.

Digital Media

Electronic or digital media has taken over print as a far less expensive option with a longer shelf life. This includes email marketing, social media, blogs, website content, and text messaging. The benefits of electronic media include immediacy and the ease of changing or updating information, production costs, and labor.

Broadcast Media

Broadcast media, such as video and audio, can be leveraged through new technology as images and sound can be conveyed online. Production devices such as video cameras have significantly decreased production costs, making this technology much easier to work with and share.

Multichannel Campaigns Can Drive More Engagement

Consumers are actively engaged across numerous channels and devices which make multichannel campaigns a feasible choice. With a multichannel campaign, brands, products, and services will have more presence across different channels.

Creating a coherent message across several channels allows you to remind your database of current patients and clients about what you offer to build brand awareness and stimulate them toward conversion.

In this environment, some consumers won't respond to display ads, but hearing an ad through programmatic audio might capture their attention. A multichannel campaign helps to guide you to the channels and formats that will work best for your select target audience.

Multichannel campaigns cover the entire funnel by creating multiple points of contact for the target audience. This offers more opportunities for acquisition.

When building a multichannel strategy, social media and video can be used effectively to drive awareness. Continued exposure to your brand across various channels and devices can help drive users further into the funnel, toward conversion.

With so many marketing channels to decipher, it can be challenging to determine which ones will be most effective to drive more clients to your practice.

With the right mix of channels, you can reach users at all touch points throughout their journey.

Multichannel campaigns are an opportunity to capture users throughout the entire marketing funnel, allowing advertisers to build awareness and consideration which leads to purchases. This will enable your marketing team to design campaigns around customer journeys, reach people at different stages throughout their journeys, and stay relevant for when they are ready to pull the trigger and sign up for a service or product.

Using a variety of tools can help deliver messages to more than one group of audiences. Combining traditional tools, such as digital newsletters, emails, social channels, video, text messaging can help to get your message across to a much wider audience. Search Engine Optimization (SEO) is used to improve your website's visibility in search engine results. It is a long-term strategy that requires constant attention and a reasonable budget, but it can be very effective at driving leads to your practice or medspa.

Although some of your audiences may have different communication preferences, there will always be some common ground.

For example, if your target audiences sweep across a wide range from Gen Y to their moms and grandmothers, it may be wise to create marketing content that can be effective for two groups. You can consider breaking each demographic into groups of up to age 35 and then 36 plus, if that makes sense for your demographic. The alternative could be dividing your database by treatment history instead of age group.

Caveat: *Be careful not to alienate your loyal, older patients or clients in favor of catering to Gen X and Z. Ideally, your bottom line will fare better if you can keep both demographics in your practice.*

Value of Text Messaging

Adding text messaging to your marketing plan is nearly essential in most markets now.

These short message services, limited to 160 characters, are appealing because they are immediate and can be sent to anyone with a cell phone. As far as I am aware, every mobile network supports SMS.

Multimedia message services (MMS) have greatly improved as they are getting more popular with retailers, pharmacies, doctors, and every other business we interact with on a daily basis.

We live on our mobile devices 24/7, so it's natural for consumers to warm up to the idea of hearing from an aesthetic physician's office via text, too, especially for routine communications, such as appointment reminders and prescription renewals. It may help to promote loyalty to your practice and cut down on cancellations and no-shows.

However, your data and patients' medical records need to be secure, and your communications must be encrypted before they ever get transferred. Encrypted messages can only be read by the intended recipient. Even if your message gets intercepted during the exchange, it would still be safe and protected from spying eyes.

Be sure to download an app or subscribe to a platform that offers services for encrypting your data before you send it through normal, unsafe channels. Search for "secure messaging solutions" to find out what is available for IOS and Android devices in your market.

Text messaging has emerged as a must-have marketing tactic. The question is not whether you should implement this system in your business, but rather how best to do it. Consumers have grown accustomed to getting messages from all or most of the service businesses they deal with. It is an efficient and affordable way to get your message across in a timely manner, and to stay top of mind to customers or patients who already know you.

The Ins and Outs of Text Messaging

- Nail the subject line to catch the reader's attention so they want to read more.
- Every word and image counts. You're competing with a steady stream of messages in consumers' inboxes.
- To get more eyes on your content, keep it short, sweet, and upbeat in tone.
- Remember to include contact information to get a response.
- Before you make a call, ask for permission to avoid getting blocked.
- Doublecheck auto correct to avoid your messages getting distorted.
- Remember that it's hard to convey emotions via texts so avoid verbiage that may be misread.
- Never use all caps. It may come across like you're angry or screaming.
- Succinct messages are easier to read, understand, and reply to.
- Avoid emojis and abbreviations – they may come across as unprofessional and not serious.
- Include a call to action in your message so recipients can take the next step; such as text, call, come in, bring a friend, etc.

Examples of Text Message CTAs

- *Create your VIP account today and take 15% off your first skincare purchase.*
- *Susan, Blue Moon Spa is offering a 3 for 2 special on our signature RF Microneeding series to our preferred clients. Want in?*
- *Someone told us it was your birthday Rachel !! Enjoy 20% off your favorite treatment to celebrate your special day from your friends at XYZ Spa. Terms apply.*

What Platforms Have the Highest ROI

Check out these top five marketing trends according to HubSpot.

The top 5 marketing trends with the highest ROI are shown in Figure 8.3.

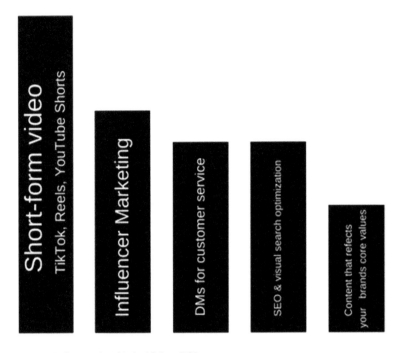

FIGURE 8.3   Top 5 marketing trends with the highest ROI

TIPS FOR SUCCESSFUL TEXT MESSAGING

1. Get written consent before sending texts to patients or clients.
2. Avoid spam words in your content so your texts don't get deleted or flagged.
3. Identify your name & business so the recipient knows who is sending the text and doesn't opt out.
4. Personalized campaigns for individual patients and groups of patients are more effective than generic, overly salesy texts.
5. Use a service or assign staff to respond to texts promptly.
6. Adding a little humor can be helpful to engage recipients – keep it light.
7. Let clients and patients know how to opt in to your SMS offers.
8. Use texts to confirm appointments, allow recipients to confirm, cancel, and reschedule.
9. Don't bombard the same clients with too many texts or texts that are not relevant to them.
10. Honor requests for opting out promptly and invite them to come back any time.

9

Future Proof Your Practice With AI

The future depends on what you do today.

Mahatma Gandhi

In today's world, marketing strategies are rapidly changing, especially in the new era of AI and everything it brings to the table.

To stay lean, mean, and profitable, think about how your business can stay relevant and keep engaging your target audiences.

The Impact of Voice Technology

The use of voice assistants, and voice technology more generally, has been on the rise over the past few years thanks, in part, to the rapid consumer adoption of smart speakers and devices.

However, the pandemic made it clear that voice technology has now become imperative where it was once simply considered a "nice-to-have" addition to medical practices. For businesses and workplaces, the implementation of voice technology is no longer a novelty. Rather, it has advanced customer service and facilitates great strides towards improved efficiency that patients appreciate.

Chatbots and Virtual Assistants

Perhaps in part due to the pandemic, voice assistants have been steadily proliferating as more consumers seek to avoid as much human interaction as possible.

For example, contactless chip card payments are seeing unprecedented rates of adoption. Kiosks powered by voice technology are popping up in places like airports, limited-service restaurants, mass transit hubs, and high-traffic retailers. Stores using technologies like Apple Pay, Samsung Pay, Google Pay, and other contactless transaction options are everywhere now.

There also seems to be a tremendous strain on call centers and customer service posts in stores. This has created long wait times and frustrated customers.

Enter virtual assistants to fill the gap. Chatbots and voice AIs can respond to customers 24/7 and alleviate some of the burden on call centers. Although some of us get annoyed at having to talk to a bot, wouldn't you rather try to get the info you need or book that table or flight faster rather than stay on hold for minutes to hours? Chatbots are now part of our lives and without them, customer service for all industries will take a big hit.

When human contact is not possible, a voice assistant or chatbot is the next best thing to being there. They have an important role to play in keeping us connected and getting our queries or problems resolved.

The newest frontier in patient communications is voice-activated search. I often refer to Alexa and Siri as my "employees of the month." I sometimes unwittingly say "thank you" when they complete a task for me, which speaks to the fact that the more you use them, the more 'human' they become.

DOI: 10.1201/9780429356742-9

DID YOU KNOW THAT WE CAN SPEAK THREE TIMES FASTER THAN WE CAN TYPE?

According to a study from Stanford University, for the English language, speech recognition was three times faster than typing, and the error rate was 20.4% lower. (https://news.stanford.edu/2016/08/24/stanford-study-speech-recognition-faster-texting)

Efficiency is the most cited reason people use voice search. As technology continues to advance, voice will expand its important role in every facet of our lives. For example, more people are using voice assistants to look for local businesses. So, if people say "lip fillers near me," you want your practice to show up on their phones.

We have learned how to speak our commands and get things done instantly. This cuts down on the time it takes to accomplish most tasks, which leaves more time to do the things you enjoy, like taking your kids to the park or working out.

Choose the Key Metrics for Your Main Objectives

- *What is your target audience?*
- *Define your secondary audience.*
- *How are they using voice search now?*
- *What words and phrases are clients most likely to be searching for to find your practice or medspa?*
- *How can you convert people who are searching for what you offer to become real, aka 'paying patients'?*

This will vary depending on the country, city, and even postcode where you practice. For example, if you cater to a more mature demographic, they may not be as comfortable with technology as Gen Z, but they will get there soon.

The instant gratification generation (Gen Z and Y) expects their needs to be met or preferably exceeded instantly and efficiently. Voice search has taken it to a whole new level!

Most voice searches are used by mobile users, so your site first needs to be SEO optimized for your local market to receive considerable "citations" as a "trusted" source for search engines to bring up. You can also optimize your local business for discovery via brand and knowledge voice search queries.

SEO for voice is pretty much like SEO for any search. The main difference is that you need to create content that will be able to talk back. Consider how a consumer in your target demographic may search for your practice and use the same words or cadence to reach them.

Introducing Chatbots to Your Practice

Chatbots have emerged as an essential component of a modern and functional website, and a must-have AI application for all businesses. They provide support and assistance 24/7 to increase customer satisfaction and reduce response time when your business is closed. They are much more cost-effective than a call center.

The technology is constantly improving to be more sophisticated and personalized, giving each customer a different experience. For example, they can be programmed for your specific needs to ask customers what they need help with and share a list of options to choose from.

The next generation of chatbots will offer more customization that will take their capabilities from the basics to providing visitors with specific answers to questions about procedures and scheduling.

Consumers are now acclimated to dealing with chatbots from a wide range of businesses they deal with every day. Customize what your chatbot can say and do to continually keep up with patient demands.

Start with basic tasks, such as, "Where are you located?" or "Is there parking nearby?" and go from there.

As you get accustomed to it, create more complex responses for your chatbot to help with, such as:

- *I need to change (or cancel) my appointment*
- *Do you take insurance and which ones?*
- *Do you offer (specific treatment) or (skincare brand)?*
- *When is the next appointment available?*
- *Is there a fee for a consultation?*
- *What days do you see clients?*
- *Can I get laser hair removal in your clinic?*
- *Does Nurse Jane do lip fillers?*
- *Do you have HydraFacial?*

Take it to the next level by getting more granular.

Think of it this way: Programming an intelligent chatbot is like having your office open 24/7 for current clients and prospective clients to get answers to everything from simple to more specific queries, depending on how sophisticated your bot has been programmed. They can also be programmed to respond to specific queries with next-generation systems that continue to get more sophisticated by offering smarter options to tap into.

There is really no limit to what chatbots can do. The myriad of benefits far exceeds the reasonable costs that are involved in setting up a system for your practice or medspa.

Cross Over to the Age of AI

In 2015, OpenAI started out as an artificial intelligence research company founded by Silicon Valley investors (Elon Musk et al.) and quickly went from a non-profit to a for-profit entity, as these things tend to go. Released on November 30, 2022, ChatGPT is credited with being the first model of this technology. From where I sit, it has dominated the category until 2023 when AI really took off.

Of course, as one would expect, a plethora of Silicon Valley techies and elsewhere jumped on board in record time to get their piece of this powerful and potentially life-changing trend.

OpenAI is a natural language processing tool driven by AI technology that allows you to have human-like conversations and much more with a chatbot. The language model can answer questions and assist with tasks such as composing emails, essays, and code.

What is does:

ChatGPT allows users to type natural language prompts and generates copy in seconds. The important thing to keep in mind is that the copy it spits out may not be accurate and may have been curated from many sources.

- **OpenAI**: Non-profit research company founded in 2015 that aims to develop and direct artificial intelligence, or AI, to benefit humanity. Elon Musk claims to be the founder along with Sam Altman, who was warning everyone who would listen about the potential dangers of the platform.
- **ChatGPT**: OpenAI's AI-powered chatbot that uses natural language processing to create human-like conversational dialogue, respond to questions, and compose written content – including articles, social media posts, and emails – and countless more sophisticated tasks that turn up every time you log on.

"Artificial intelligence is the science of making machines do things that would require intelligence if done by men." – Marvin Minsky

Get on Board AI or Risk Extinction

At this point, all or most industries, from small businesses to global conglomerates, are now using voice search and WIFI-enabled marketing, and more continue to follow. This is the new normal, so don't get left behind!

AI quickly became a buzzword for marketers, and AI has proven to be a force to revolutionize the way all businesses approach their marketing strategies, including aesthetic practices and medspas.

AI uses algorithms and machine learning to automate tasks and make predictions based on data analysis. Thus, it can analyze consumer behavior, improve targeting, personalize content, and automate customer service, among many other important time-saving tasks.

AI can process and analyze vast amounts of data in real-time, which makes it an essential tool to tap into when promoting your services to prospective patients. The more efficient your marketing tactics are, the better results you can achieve from your efforts, which can also reduce costs and manpower.

It should come as no surprise that since ChatGPT basically changed our work, every other tech company is on a mission to get their piece of the AI pie to stay relevant.

The rapid advancement of AI has revolutionized the way we work, engage with each other and learn. AI has had a massive effect on all businesses in unlimited ways in a very short time. You cannot ignore it and the sooner you get on board, the better.

Change is welcome when it makes things better and advances what we can do. Progress is the ultimate result when change is good. The rapid advancement of AI represents a sea of change in the way we work, engage with each other and learn. It will impact everything you do from now into the future to market and grow your business.

This is not just a fleeting trend: it is coming to a device near you, whether you know it or like it or not.

ChatGPT AI Types

ChatGPT can potentially make your life easier in many ways if take the time to learn the details.

Here are some of the most relevant primary types of AI for medical practices and spas.

Each of them has unique characteristics and functions:

- **Narrow AI (or Weak AI)** systems are designed to perform specific tasks or solve specific problems within a limited domain. These systems are specialized so they can handle a single task, such as image recognition or natural language processing.
- **Machine Learning (ML)**: A cousin of AI that focuses on developing algorithms and models that enable computers to learn from data and make predictions or decisions without being explicitly programmed.
- **General AI (Strong AI)**: Works to replicate human-like intelligence and is able to understand, learn, and apply knowledge across multiple domains. END

Newsflash: Did you know that AI can be programmed to perform most or all intellectual tasks that humans can do?

Get Educated

Here are six online courses to look into to get some guidance on how to use AI ethically.

My team found some of these very helpful because you can pace yourself and log on anytime – no pressure.

CHART:

COURSERA	<u>coursera.org</u>
EDX	<u>edx.org</u>
FAST AI	<u>fast.ai</u>
TENSORFLOW	<u>tensorflow.org</u>
SUBSTACK	<u>substack.com/</u>
LINKEDIN	<u>Linkedin.com/learning/topics/</u> <u>artificial-intelligence</u>

P.S. Don't mistake 'AI' for other components of technology. For example, "machine learning" is a phrase that pops up a lot, but it is not the same as AI. It may also require specialized hardware and software for writing and training machine learning algorithms.'

According to Bing, machine learning is used today for a wide range of commercial purposes, such as suggesting products to consumers based on their past purchases, predicting stock market fluctuations, and translating text from one language to another.

AI-Powered Features in Search Engines

AI can distill complex information and multiple perspectives into easy-to-digest formats, so you can quickly understand the big picture and learn more online.

You can test the waters by generating ideas and quick research. However, before you actually use any content AI spits out, do some fact-checking to make sure it makes sense and is not plagiarized from a source that might sue you.

ChatGPT has a free version and a paid version to use its platform. The latter, called simply, ChatGPT Plus, is an upgrade. Surely there will be more paid features to tap into soon on all these platforms, just like every other discovery that originated in Silicon Valley.

In its own words, ChatGPT is "conversational AI that can chat with you, answer follow-up questions, and challenge incorrect assumptions."

To get started follow these three simple prompts:

1. Go to chat.openai.com and create an OpenAI account.
2. Sign in to start chatting with ChatGPT.
3. Start a conversation by asking a question or posting a statement.

Cool ChatGPT Tip – *Did you know you can use ChatGPT in dark mode or light mode?*
Go to the settings menu, click on the "Appearance" tab, select 'Dark Mode'

4 AI Chatbots in Order of Launch Date (as of this printing)

ChatGPT – The original AI platform that hails from Silicon Valley, founded by Elon Musk and Sam Altman as a 'research organization' in December 2015.

https://openai.com/

Who owns it – OpenAI, San Francisco, USA – and Microsoft owns 49%.

What it is – An AI-powered chatbot that uses natural language processing to create human-like conversa- tional dialogue, respond to questions, and compose written content including articles, social media posts, emails, and much more.

Costs to use – It requires an OpenAI account and a subscription to use the ChatGPT Plus upgraded version, which at the time of this printing costs $20 USD per month. It is available in most markets across the world, but not all due to government restrictions.

Features – Versions include:

ChatGPT (free)

ChatGPT Plus (paid)

 ## Bard *

Bard: Bard is Google's answer to OpenAI. It is an AI-powered chatbot that simulates human conversations using natural language processing and machine learning. It requires a Google account, and it supplements Google search.

https://bard.google.com

Who owns it – Google

What it is – AI-powered chatbot

Costs to use – Free to use if you are on Google; access it through bard.google.com and log in with your account

Features – Bard can be integrated into websites, messaging platforms, or other applications to provide natural language responses to questions.

 ## Copilot

Microsoft Copilot: Formerly known as BING Chat, now called Microsoft Copilot as of 2023, is an AI chatbot developed by Microsoft and released in 2023, based on the same technology that OpenAI uses. Microsoft "recommends" that users accept Microsoft's Edge web browser. The platform is built-in whenever you search in Microsoft Edge, otherwise, you may have to log out of your browser to get on.

copilot.microsoft.com

Who owns it – Microsoft

What it is – AI chatbot

Costs to use – You need to have a Microsoft Copilot account to load the Bing App/Microsoft Copilot to access it for free.

Features – In some markets, you may be able to choose your preferred conversational style to be more creative, more balanced, or more precise, which is kind of cool.

ANTHROP\C

Claude Pro: Still in Beta as of this printing, Claude 2 and 2.1 AI are upgraded versions of the original Claude chatbot platform. Claude 2 is referred to as a 'conversational assistant' that can help you navigate tasks and goals. Claude Pro is their answer to the paid GPT Plus model that allows you to gain **5x more usage** than their earlier model, Claude 2. The company's stated mission is: "Anthropic exists for our mission: to ensure transformative AI helps people and society flourish."

https://claude.ai/

---

* As of February 2024, Google renamed their generative AI brands as 'Gemini'.

What it is – An AI chatbot developed by Anthropic AI, a startup co-founded by former members of OpenAI.

Who owns it – Anthropic, San Francisco, USA

Costs to use – Free to date while in Beta. Pro is $20 US monthly or Eighteen Pounds Sterling in British pounds

Features – Different from some other chatbots by including learning from conversations and data, that can be adapted to different contexts and languages. I find it to be simple to use at this stage, and it feels very personal still at this stage.

ChatGPT Cheat Sheet

This platform offers a wide range of functions that you may never need to use. In addition to answering simple questions, it can compose essays, create AI prompts, have deep philosophical conversations, and much more. Its talents are only limited by your imagination. ChatGPT can even code for you if you want to go there.

The ChatGPT text box at the bottom of the page is where you type your inquiries. Start by asking easy questions to get the hang of it. OpenAI recommends inputting a statement to generate the best result.

If you aren't satisfied with the result you get, try, try, again. Use different phrasing or more simple language or formatting to get to what you want to achieve.

*Caveat: Be sure to assess the feasibility and accuracy for every recommendation AI's spit out before using them. Get a second opinion from another AI and/or use a second respected source to stay safe. ChatGPT has a disclaimer at the bottom of the site for a reason: '**ChatGPT can make mistakes. Consider checking important information.**'*

Try This Exercise

Ask ChatGPT-Plus how to make your practice more profitable in a statement rather than just a question. I used this prompt:

"make my aesthetic medical practice profitable. What strat"""What strategies can help to increase sales and attract more clients to my aesthetics practice?"

ChatGPT-Plus

To make an aesthetic medical practice more profitable and attract more clients, you might consider implementing several strategies. Here are some that are commonly effective:

1. **Enhance Online Presence**:
   - Improve your website to make it more user-friendly and informative.
   - Utilize search engine optimization (SEO) to increase your visibility on search engines.
   - Engage with clients through social media platforms by sharing before-and-after photos, client testimonials, and educational content.
2. **Leverage Digital Marketing**:
   - Use targeted online advertising to reach potential clients in your area.
   - Implement email marketing campaigns to keep in touch with existing clients and inform them of new services or promotions.
3. **Offer Competitive Pricing and Packages**:
   - Research your competitors' pricing and consider offering competitive rates.
   - Create package deals for services that clients often use together or return for regularly.

4. **Introduce a Loyalty Program**:
   - Reward repeat clients with discounts or free services after a certain number of visits or referrals.
5. **Host Educational Events**:
   - Organize seminars or webinars to educate potential clients about the services you offer and the benefits of aesthetic treatments.
6. **Improve Client Experience**:
   - Provide excellent customer service to make clients feel valued and likely to return.
   - Ensure a comfortable and inviting clinic environment.
   - Follow up with clients after procedures to check on their recovery and satisfaction.
7. **Networking with Other Professionals**:
   - Collaborate with other healthcare professionals for referrals.
   - Establish relationships with local businesses for cross-promotion.
8. **Get Client Feedback**:
   - Regularly collect client feedback to improve services and address any concerns promptly.
9. **Expand Your Service Offerings**:
   - Stay updated with the latest trends and technologies in aesthetic medicine and consider offering new and in-demand services.
10. **Invest in Training**:
   - Ensure your team is highly skilled and trained in the latest techniques to provide the best possible outcomes for clients.
11. **Monitor and Adapt**:
   - Keep an eye on your business metrics to understand where you're doing well and where there's room for improvement.
   - Be willing to adapt your strategies based on what the data is telling you.

By implementing these strategies, you can work towards increasing sales and attracting more clients to your aesthetic medical practice. It's essential to have a clear plan and continuously evaluate the effectiveness of your strategies, making adjustments as necessary.

Overall score:

I would give ChatGPT Plus a solid 7. These tips are pretty basic and not very actionable.

Next, go back and tweak your query so that you can elicit more relevant intel.

Aim for more specific tips and ideas for strategies that you can implement into your practice and

Try it a few different ways until you reach the information a

Overall score:

I would give ChatGPT Plus a solid 7.

These tips are pretty basic and not actionable enough.

Next, go back and tweak your query so that you can elicit more relevant intel.

Go for specific tips and strategies that you can implement into your practice in a reasonable time frame and measure results.

Don't give your AI too much work to do all at once or it may get confused.

Use AI as an advisor to stay on top of the meda-trends in medical aesthetics and AI

Look for resources to keep you up to speed on the most important trends that your patients and clients are interested in.

- *Loreal.com – Check out Loreal's portfolio of beauty brands and cutting-edge research on this trend*
- *perfectcorp.com – One of the early adapters to use innovative technology in the aesthetics space for patient education. END*

How is ChatGPT Different from a Search Engine

- ChatGPT is an AI language model(AKA chatbot) created to hold a conversation with the user.
- Search engines index web pages to help the user find the information they ask for.
- ChatGPT is not able to search the internet for information. It uses the information it learned from training data to generate a response, which may not always be accurate.
- ChatGPT is not exactly an encyclopedia of everything you want to know. In fact, it doesn't really have any specific kind of knowledge.

Navigating Prompt Engineering

Anyone can type anything into AI, but getting good results requires an understanding of how to choose and use prompts. "Prompts" is short for "prompt engineering."

Learning how to use the right prompts is a critical success factor if you want to master your AI skills. After all, you are interacting with a robot that doesn't have a brain and didn't go to Harvard.

This is one of the most important key learnings for AI. Although you may be able to get what you need by using simple prompts, the quality of results you achieve is dependent on how much information you provide the AI and how well it is crafted. It sounds simple and straightforward on the surface, but it is not even close.

A prompt may contain information like the instruction or question you are passing to the model and include other details such as context, inputs, or examples. You need to use these elements to instruct the AI in the best possible way to generate the specific results you need.

Don't presume that you can get it right on the first few tries. After playing with this for a bit, you will get the hang of the concept and get better over time. In the meantime, we can expect that the AI community will continue to make these tasks easier for regular people, i.e., not engineers.

Mastering how to use prompts will help you get the most out of your AI experience. The more concise and on-point your prompts are, the better responses you can get from the technology. A prompt may contain information such as a question you want to pose with additional details in terms of context, inputs, or examples.

By using the right prompts, you will reap the benefit of better results with greater specifics faster.

Don't despair! It may take a few lessons, a course or two, and a lot of trial and error to master the tasks you need to use AI platforms. It is a new way of working that has great rewards and is worth the effort to master it.

Eight AI Tools You Can Use

Note: Most of these are paid, but some are free.

1 Wordtune	Offers text improvements as you write	https://app.wordtune.com
2 Jasper	Brand content creator	https://www.jasper.ai
3 Chatgptwriter	Helps to write emails and messages fast	https://chatgptwriter.ai
4 Chat Prompt Genius	Generates prompts and content ideas for chatbot conversations	https://chatpromptgenius.com/
5 Kaleido	Removes backgrounds from images and videos	https://www.kaleido.ai/products
6 PDF.ai	Chat with any document	https://pdf.ai
7 Rose.ai	Fast way to do research	https://rose.ai/
8 Aivalley.ai	Source of AI prompts & tools	https://aivalley.ai/

Google's Gemini

Google joined the AI party in January 2023 with Gemini. It is integrated into Google's search engine to enhance their responses to queries, which comes in very handy for Google users. This chatbot's raison d'etre is to simplify complex topics in a way that can be easily understood by anyone, from a child to an octogenarian.

Chat GPT and Gemini are both LLMs that translate loosely to a massive database of text data that can generate "human-like" responses to your prompts. The text comes from a wide range of sources which can add up to billions or trillions of words by now.

Accuracy: Gemini is designed to be as accurate as possible. It is trained on a dataset of text that has been carefully curated to ensure that it is accurate and factual. ChatGPT is not as focused on accuracy as Gemini. It is trained on a dataset of text that includes both accurate and inaccurate information. This means that ChatGPT may sometimes provide inaccurate information, while Gemini is more likely to provide accurate information.

Creativity: Gemini is capable of generating creative material, such as stories, and code. ChatGPT is also capable of generating creative text, but it is not as good at it as Gemini. Gemini is able to generate more creative text because it is trained on a dataset of text that includes both creative and non-creative text. ChatGPT is trained on a dataset of text that is mostly non-creative.

Interface: Gemini is available through the Google Assistant and the Google Search website. ChatGPT is available through the OpenAI website. Gemini's interface is more user-friendly than ChatGPT's interface. Gemini's interface is also more integrated with other Google products, such as Gmail and Google Docs.

Gemini and ChatGPT are both powerful tools that can be used for a variety of purposes. However, there are some key differences between these platforms that may make nictitate using both or more (Figure 9.1).

12 STEPS TO JOIN SUBSTACK – Ready to take the plunge?

This popular platform is flooded with tech topics from experts, and growing

1. Go to Substack.com, click "Start writing", and go through the prompts to create an account
2. Pick a title, URL, logo, and short description of yourself
3. Customize your theme - who you are, what you do, etc.

Feature	Bard	ChatGPT
Data source	Massive dataset of text and code	Dataset of text and code that is updated more frequently
Accuracy	Designed to be as accurate as possible	Not as focused on accuracy as Bard
Creativity	Capable of generating creative text	Capable of generating creative text, but not as good as Bard
Interface	Available through the Google Assistant and the Google Search website	Available through the OpenAI website
Best for	People who need accurate and creative text	People who need up-to-date information and creative text

FIGURE 9.1   Gemini (Formerly BARD) vs. ChatGPT

4. Setup your about page, emails, unsubscribe page, banners, headers, footers
5. Readers can sign up for a Substack as a free or paying reader
6. Feel things out and build an audience by tapping into other relevant writers' content
7. Before you hit publish, send a copy to yourself to see what it looks like and check your spelling
8. Add calls-to-action to posts to encourage readers to subscribe, comment, and share
9. Link Substack to your website, social media, email signature, LinkedIn, etc.
10. Share your articles on social media and other platforms
11. Comment on other writers' posts to get known
12. Check the Substack Dashboard to see how you're doing

What's Coming Next?

AI is still in its infancy, but the future looks bright and exciting.

It's too late to wave a white flag about the potential pitfalls of the technology. It clearly needs to regulated in some ways by the tech community, and most likely individual governments. My hope is that this emphasis on fine-tuning and adding responsible guard rails will be widely accepted by current AI chatbots, as well as those that have yet to be created.

Looking Ahead

New developments in AI may be able to put in just a little information about your brand, and then chatbots can spit out a slew of ideas for content. You could then be able to drag and drop the ones you want to try. I am open to anything that will improve our productivity and increase accuracy, while potentially lightening our workload.

Many platforms have integrated their own versions of augmented reality and are all over this development. For example, check out Canva and see what pops up on your screen. The site is a perennial favorite around the world for creating everything you need for gorgeous graphics, invitations, social posts, charts, posters, and much more. They jumped on AI early and included Magic Write®. I keep it open on my desktop 24/7, and suggest you do the same.

The flip side of doing good with this technology, has to do with the platforms, as well as how you use it. Be transparent to patients about how you may be using AI in your practice or medspa to keep your clients

8 AI POWERED TIME SAVERS

Brandsnap	Describe your business and AI will suggest a unique name for it	brandsnap.ai
Eightify	Chrome extension for YouTube summaries powered by ChatGPT.	eightify.app
Adobe Firefly	AI powered tool to create images with text prompts	adobe.com/sensei/ge nerative-ai/firefly.html
Lovo	Realistic text-to-speech generator	lovo.ai
Alpha	Ask about historical info and market data	alphaa.ai
Gamma.ai	ChatGPT for presentations	gamma.ai
Cohesive	Customize AI templates for most types of content	cohesive.so
Monic	Learn anything academic 10x faster	/beta.monic.ai

FIGURE 9.2

in the loop. You may find that some of your older patients, who are not as tech-savvy, may find it challenging. It that is the case, it may be wise to have a Plan B to accommodate them; i.e phones and emails.

These tools will be soon be implemented in all aspects of marketing, management, content creation, interactive content, and much more. As business owners, it is important to pay careful attention to these innovations and stay ahead of the curve.

See Figure 9.2 above for 8 AI-powered time savers.

Eight Ways to Use AI in Your Marketing Plan

1. **Analytics**: AI-powered analytics can help to anticipate customer behavior and tailor the most effective marketing strategies to reach them, which can optimize your marketing strategies and improve ROI.
2. **Create better content faster**: AI-powered content creation tools can generate good content in seconds which can save time, improve the quality of your content, and enhance engagement with potential clients and patients.
3. **Image and voice recognition**: AI-powered image and voice recognition technology can help analyze your preferences and behavior through feedback, reviews, and other data sources. It can identify trends to help you design marketing strategies.
4. **Personalization**: AI can help to personalize marketing campaigns by analyzing consumer data and behavior and offering customized recommendations based on individual preferences and past purchases.
5. **Learning**: AI programming creates rules (called algorithms) for how to turn it into actionable information.
6. **Self-correction**: This aspect of AI programming is designed to continually fine-tune algorithms and ensure they provide the most accurate results.

7. **Reasoning**: This aspect of AI programming focuses on choosing the right algorithm to reach a desired outcome.
8. **Creativity**: This refers to "neural networks," or statistical methods and other AI techniques that can generate new images, text, music, and fresh ideas.

Sources: ChatGPT Plus, Bing, Microsoft

Artificial intelligence (AI) is rapidly changing the way businesses operate. From automating tasks to providing insights into customer behavior, AI is having a major impact on all businesses.

3 NEXT FRONTIERS FOR USING AI IN BUSINESS:

- *Generative AI: Generative AI can create new content, such as text, images, and music. It has the potential to revolutionize the way you create and market products and services. For example, to create personalized marketing materials or generate new ideas for events and promotions.*
- *Self-learning AI: This technology has the potential to automate many tasks that are done by humans, such as customer service. Thus, it can help you save time and money, save time and money, and upgrade your products and services.*
- *Edge AI: This type of AI can run on devices, such as iPhones and sensors, instead of in the cloud which can improve AI performance and security. It may also be used to react to fraud detection to improve the accuracy of medical diagnosis in real-time.*

These are destined to affect medical aesthetics in a big way. We just don't know how soon and how much, but it looks very promising.

Implementing AI in your business helps you work faster, better, cheaper, and more efficiently. We already know that AI has the potential to revolutionize the way you operate your business. Embracing it now gives you a competitive edge in your community.

Pivot to Stay Relevant

It's too vast to predict what AI will look like in 3 years, 5 years, etc. The field is too vast to predict exactly how this technology will evolve, and it gets more sophisticated constantly.

AI has clearly demonstrated the potential to revolutionize the way all businesses operate. This includes numerous aspects of medicine, from hospitals to aesthetic practices, and med-spas.

It is possible that AR will bring people closer and present exciting opportunities for doing business and attracting new clients. These changes are coming at us very quickly, which makes it hard to keep up with the best options for your business.

Failing to get on board with AI and everything related to this new way of communicating and reaching patients and clients is not an option anymore. Customer-focused brands and companies, including aesthetic medicine and spa services, have a lot to gain from these new tools. The next frontier for AI is predicted to be more personalized and able to offer specific applications for individual businesses. Keep an eye out for social media content generation tools coming soon to a bot near you.

The digital world is changing rapidly, and social media is a big part of it. From what I have read, it is widely accepted that VR will have a profound effect on the social media environment. Social media plat- forms will need to pivot to adopt these changes to their best advantage. Many platforms are now includ- ing AR-based advertising options that can bring more interaction and raise post engagements. Content for social media may inevitably be delivered in a 3D format powered by AR.

These developments will ultimately allow aesthetic practices and medspas to better understand their patients, and how to get to their target audiences. It may also guide partitioners to offer the right products and services at the right time to a more defined group of patients and clients. The advantages will surely be numerous.

As busy professionals, it is clearly impossible to keep up with all of the nuisances of this vastly changing field. Here, I share some of my favorite resources who are on the cutting edge of the field and may be helpful.

- CHART: My Go-To Tech Resources

My select list of the pros I follow for up-to-the-minute intel on AI.

These are Regrettably, these are all subscriptions (sorry), but you can aYou can also find these and more tech gurus who are prolific on X *formally Twitter.

*   https://apnews.com/article/ai-act-artificial-intelligence-europe-regulation-94e2b38703b38fdbfab c9580f845ef9a

1. On Tech: AI Newsletter: *New York Times* – https://www.nytimes.com/newsletters/signup/OT
2. Michael Spencer: *Artificial Intelligence Survey* – https://futuresin.substack.com
3. Kara Swisher: *New York Times* – https://www.nytimes.com/column/kara-swisher
4. Naimi Knicks: *Washington Post* – https://www.washingtonpost.com/technology/2023/06/09/meta-morale-artificial-intelligence/
5. Pranshu Verma: *Washington Post* – https://www.washingtonpost.com/people/pranshu-verma/
6. Cade Netz: *New York Times* - https://www.nytimes.com/by/cade-metz

Future Challenges and Opportunities

'AI replacing human jobs completely might be a far-fetched thought, but people who have mastered AI can easily replace your job.'
Aashray Parikh on Medium

The medical aesthetics industry is in a state of flux with changes and new ways of thinking coming at us from every direction. I see this positively as new ways of thinking tend to bring new and innovative opportunities.

We are still in the early days of AI, at least for those of us who are not MIT grads.

As AI technology continues to evolve, it will surely weave its way into our work and personal lives full stop. These tools will soon become an essential aspect of digital marketing and take over many tasks that previously required humans.

Although I am fascinated with this new frontier emerging at record speed, the potential for errors, fake news, scams, and fraudsters is a big concern. My plan is to get hyper-educated on the good, bad, and scary aspects of AI, and closely follow the trends and changes that are coming at us from all directions. As with everything new, it is probably wise to be suspicious and resistant to some of these developments.

As a business owner or practitioner, you need to be mindful of these quickly evolving trends because your patients and clients are, and your colleagues, vendors, and partners will be too. If you want to stay one step ahead of the competition, you can't hide under the bed!

For all the naysayers who think AI is just another money-making scheme from Silicon Valley, you may be putting your business at risk by not paying attention. Despite some pending regulations, it is here to stay.

We can't put the genie back in the bottle, so watch this space!

Appendix

Sample Social Media Manager Job Description

We are a fast-paced, innovative, aesthetics practice with a devoted team of talented professionals who are passionate about helping others achieve their goals. We are looking for a team player who is highly motivated, energetic, disciplined, and who can grow with us.

We have an opportunity for a Social Media Marketing Manager who will lead the overall strategy and direction of social media marketing, including but not limited to Facebook, Instagram, Twitter, YouTube, TikTok, Snap, and LinkedIn. The Social Media Marketing Manager must be experienced in social media platforms and up to date with AI trends.

The position includes working across teams to drive business needs and objectives and overseeing that KPIs are met. Being a great collaborator is important.

Job Responsibilities

- Oversee day-to-day management of campaigns and ensure brand consistency.
- Facilitate scaling brand and company awareness through various social media channels.
- Manage the implementation of a social media strategy to ensure alignment with business goals.
- Own and build out social media content publishing calendar for planning, publishing, and reporting purposes.
- Manage editing and approvals of all posts to go live, including original text, photos, videos, and news across social channels.
- Create actionable plans to grow and maintain followers on all relevant platforms.
- Monitor social channels to pick up relevant trending topics to participate in.
- Write social media copy in real-time and for future content to be used across channels.
- Collaborate and propose engaging social content to promote our brand (memes, Instagram Stories/Reels, TikTok videos) based on trends and key learnings from past initiatives.
- Assist in social quarterly campaign execution to ensure that content is organized, planned, placed, and updated appropriately.
- Work with external vendors as needed to produce campaigns and initiatives.
- Manage influencer and creator activations by identifying agency partners, vetting talent, collaborating with key stakeholders, and maintaining strategy alignment.
- Capture in-studio photography and video content to be used across social channels.
- Work in partnership with practice staff to identify engagement opportunities via social to ignite the right conversations and opportunities for the brand.

Skills and Requirements

- 5+ years of social media experience.
- BA/BS degree in Communications, Media, Public Relations, or Marketing preferred.
- Experience managing cross-functional marketing communications/PR and social media campaigns.

- Strong networking, relationship-building, interpersonal, and problem-solving skills.
- Excellent writing and presentation skills, ability to use creative tools like Canva.
- Strong attention to detail.
- Knowledge of emerging social media platforms including Instagram, Twitter, TikTok, etc.
- Expertise on where the landscape of social networking is heading and how to take advantage of the trends.
- Basic analytical skills through social reporting, identifying trends, and providing recommendations.
- Ability to work in a fast-paced environment and multi-task.
- Familiarity with social media listening tools.
- Experience in Medical Aesthetics industry is a plus.

Seniority Level

Mid-senior level

Industry Background

- Healthcare.
- Aesthetics.
- Spa.
- Salons.

Employment Type

Full-time.
  Work from home up to 25% if requested.

Job Functions

- Marketing.
- Writing.
- Creative development.

Glossary of Marketing and
AI Terms for Aesthetic Businesses

A/B Testing: Comparing two variations of a single concept or design to determine which performs best to improve the results of a marketing tactic. Often used for email marketing, calls-to-action, landing pages, ad strategies, etc.

Above the Fold: Refers to the area on a page of a website that is visible when the page loads. Therefore, it is what visitors see first and spend the most time on, so the most important content should ideally be posted there.

Advertorial: A short feature story written to appear as though it is a magazine or newspaper article, that is used as a persuasive B2B communication tactic promoting a product or sharing information about your business.

Affiliate Program: An agreement by which a business pays another business or influencer a commission for sending traffic or sales to them, typically through social media channels.

AI Prompt: Text that is used to ask a question or get information from AI.

Algorithm: An algorithm is a set of rules or calculations used to solve problems and deliver a result. Algorithms are also used in social media to deliver content to the user.

API (Application Programming Interface): A type of software interface that facilitates two or more computer programs to communicate with each other.

App: Abbreviation for an "application" that performs a specific function and is usually downloaded to a mobile device, smart phone, tablet, or watch.

Analytics: Allow marketers to assess the return on investment (ROI) of specific campaigns or tactics, such as a series of blog articles or a Google ad campaign. Analytics may include specific marketing metrics, such as conversion rate, click-through rate, marketing spend per customer, etc.

Artificial Intelligence (AI): Artificial intelligence is the ability of computers, programs, or machines to learn and adapt in ways that resemble human thinking. Chatbots use AI to communicate and answer questions. The more you interact with an AI program, the more "intelligent" it becomes, and the more data it has to work with.

Artificial Neural Networks (ANNs): These networks can absorb vast amounts of input data and process it through multiple layers that extract and learn the data's features.

Auto Response: A response programmed to be sent automatically to incoming messages (such as emails, out of office messages, etc.).

Avatar: An avatar is a visual representation of a person used in digital media, typically a computer-generated image. The term "avatar" may also refer to a photo posted in profiles on social channels, or a company logo used for that purpose.

B2B (Business-to-Business): Used to describe brands, businesses, or tactics that are designed to reach other businesses.

B2B (Business-to-Consumer): Used to describe brands, businesses, or tactics that are designed to reach consumers.

Backlinks: A backlink is defined as when one website gets linked to another with anchor text.

Bard: Google Bard is an AI-powered chatbot designed to simulate human conversations using natural language processing and machine learning.

Big Data: Datasets that are too big or complex to be used by traditional data processing methods.

Bing: The AI chatbot integrated into Microsoft's Bing search engine.

Bitly: Free URL shortener plus link management software, QR Code features, and Link-in-bio solutions.

Blue Checkmark: A blue checkmark (or blue check or blue tick) is a symbol used on many social media platforms to indicate that an account's identity has been verified. Verification is usually reserved for accounts that are most likely to be targeted by copycats, like celebrities, brands, or influencers.

Bottom of the Funnel (BoFu): The final stage of a client or patient's experience with a brand or practice when they are ready to take the next step, such as requesting a sample or having a consultation.

Bounce Rate: The percentage of targets that land on a page on your website or receive an email and then leave without clicking or taking any action. A high bounce rate usually means poor conversion rates because visitors are not staying long enough to engage.

Branding: The strategic process used to influence the perception of products or services in the market. This may include logos, color schemes, imagery, mission statements, and any other marketing tactics that represent a business or person.

Buyer Persona: Buyer personas are created to identify the demographic, psychographic, and behavioral information of the ideal customers for a product or brand.

Call-to-action (CTA): A call-to-action is a specific phrase used on marketing collateral that directs customers to perform a specific action. Calls-to-action might include "Buy Now," "Book a Call," "Download a Free PDF," or "Add to Cart."

CAN-SPAM: Stands for "Controlling the Assault of Non-Solicited Pornography and Marketing," a US law that establishes the rules for commercial email and commercial messages. It gives recipients the right to have a business stop emailing. Penalties attach for anyone who violates the law. Other countries may have similar regulations, such as CASL, "Canadian Anti-Spam Legislation."

Chatbot: A chatbot is a type of bot that uses artificial intelligence to answer questions and perform simple tasks in messaging apps such as Facebook Messenger. These are commonly used for customer service, data and lead collection, purchasing recommendations, appointments, etc.

ChatGPT: GPT stands for "generative pre-trained transformer." It was the first AI-based chatbot launched by OpenAI in 2022.

Churn Rate: Represents the number of clients or patients who stop having services or buying products over a specific period. This is calculated by dividing the number of clients lost during a set period by the total number of clients the business had at the beginning of that period.

Clickthrough Rate (CTR): The number of clicks your ad receives divided by the number of times your ad is shown; clicks ÷ impressions = CTR.

Co-Branding: A collaboration between two brands to promote each other's products and services. The main advantage is that each brand is exposed to a new customer base.

Code Generator: Software techniques or systems that generate program code which can be used independently of the generator system.

Conversion Rate: Conversion rate is the number of conversions divided by the number of visitors. It is a metric that allows you to measure how well your marketing efforts are working to achieve specific goals.

Content Management System (CMS): Software that is utilized to hold contact information and other records related to a specific lead, contact, or business, typically used by sales professionals to track their interactions and status.

Creators: Creators are professionals who create original content in many forms including digital, video, photos, and graphics to post online. They are typically hired and paid for their work. The most popular sites include TikTok, Instagram, and YouTube.

Customer Acquisition Cost (CAC): The amount needed to acquire a new customer or client who purchases a product or service.

Customer Relationship Management (CRM): Customer relationship management (CRM) encompasses all aspects of technology used to manage relationships with customers. CRM involves data from multiple touchpoints in the customer lifecycle, including data that is generated from sales, marketing, customer service, etc.

Customer Retention: Any type of action or strategy taken to ensure that existing customers or clients continue to come back to your practice and stay loyal. Customer retention rate measures the number of customers retained for a specific period.

Dall-E: AI system from ChatGPT that can create realistic images and art from a description in natural language.

Data Mining: A way to discover patterns in large data sets involving machine learning, statistics, and databases.

Data Set: Collection of related data points, usually with a uniform order and tags.

Deep Learning: A subset of machine learning that uses deep neural networks, layers of connected "neurons" whose connections have parameters, or weights that can be trained. Used for learning from unstructured data such as images, text, and audio.

DEI: Diversity, equity, and inclusion (DEI) are decisive calls-to-action that businesses need to Be up to date on and incorporate, at least in markets like the US and the UK. Making an effort to promote diversity, equity, and inclusion is an important concept to pay attention to, or you may get called out on social media channels.

Direct Message (DM): Private message sent via social media platforms between two or more users. Certain platforms limit direct messages to users who follow you.

E-book: An e-book is a digitized book that is often used for lead generation, providing useful information in a concise format. Users fill out a form with personal information to be able to download the e-book.

Earned Media: As opposed to paid media, earned media is organic content that may be picked up by news outlets, bloggers, magazines, or others and appears online or in print without having to incur any costs.

Engagement Rate: The rate at which audience members or followers are actively interacting with social media content, such as commenting on a post or sharing a Tweet. Rates can be measured by engagement rate per post, by reach, and by impression.

Evergreen Content: Evergreen content has a long lifespan. It stays relevant and fresh, no matter the publication or distribution date.

Feed: An updated list of all the new content posted by the accounts a user follows on social media, usually controlled by an algorithm.

GDPR: Stands for "General Data Protection Regulation." This is an EU law that sets the standards for data protection and privacy and monitors the way personal information is used.

Gen X: Generation X follows the baby boomer generation and precedes the millennial generation. Typically used to describe the generation born between 1965 and 1980.

Gen Y: Generation Y, also known as digital natives or millennials, were born between 1981 and 1996.

Gen Z: Members of Generation Z were born after 1995.

Generative AI: This term refers to any automated process that uses algorithms to produce new data – the operative word being "new." Also called Strong AI.

Geotargeting: The practice of targeting visitors online with localized or location-appropriate content based on a visitor's geographic location.

GIF: GIF is an acronym for "graphics interchange format," which is a file format that supports both static and animated images.

Gift With Purchase (GWP): A marketing tactic used to attract customers and increase the average order through a purchase-with-purchase promotion that rewards the buyer for making a purchase by offering a second product at a discounted price if bought together.

GoogleMyBusiness: Free business profile that appears on Google Search and Google Maps to attract customers. You can personalize your profile with photos, offers, posts, etc.

Graphics Processing Units (GPUs): Computer chips originally developed for use in video games that are also used for deep learning applications. In contrast, traditional machine learning and other analyses usually run on central processing units (CPUs) or a computer's processor.

Hashtag: A metadata tag using the hash symbol (#) before a word or phrase. Hashtags allow users to cross-reference their content across social media platforms, such as an Instagram post or a Tweet. Branded hashtags are unique to the user.

HIPAA: Stands for "Health Insurance Portability and Accountability Act," a US federal law that strictly regulates privacy and security for patients. All healthcare professionals must comply with HIPAA standards.

HTML: Stands for "hypertext markup language," and is the standard language used for displaying content retrieved from the internet.

Impressions: Impressions or an impression is a metric used to measure the number of times your post has been seen on social media.

Inbound Marketing: Inbound marketing uses blogs, social media, and SEO to attract customers through the most relevant and useful content.

Influencer: An individual who has a loyal following and engaged audience on social platforms. They are often used by marketers and brands as part of a paid partnership or campaign to promote a product or brand to their followers.

Infographic: Using images and data in the form of bar graphs, pie charts, line graphs, and tables to tell a story or present a topic to the user.

Instagram Bio Link: "Link-in-bio" refers to the clickable URL that you can add to your profile section.

Key Performance Indicators (KPIs): Key Performance Indicators (KPIs) are metrics that a business uses to measure engagement, profit, sales, satisfaction, or another area of performance. KPIs specific to marketing include Customer Acquisition Cost (CAC), Customer Lifetime Value (LTV), and conversion rate.

Landing Pages: Landing pages may include your website, blog, or other digital real estate where you want to direct traffic. These are implemented to direct your audience to engage with specific messaging for something you want to promote, such as information about a new product or treatment, special offers, events, podcasts, or clinic news.

Large Language Model (LLM): An LLM is a massive database of text data that comes from a wide range of sources and can be referenced to generate human-like responses to prompts.

Leads: Leads are potential customers who have actively engaged with content or marketing materials, and therefore have entered the marketing funnel. Lead nurturing refers to driving them toward a sale or other engagement through marketing tactics and other forms of communication. Lead generation is the cost of getting a new customer.

Lifetime Value of a Client (LTV): This exercise is designed to help predict the net profit attributed to your future relationship with a customer based on the revenue paid in a perspective time period.

Listicle: An article or content that is written in a list format, such as "10 Best Listicles of 2023," often used for social media content.

Live Chat: A tool that connects customers with actual, human support representatives. This allows your users to resolve issues in real-time.

Logo: A symbol compromised of words, images, and colors that is used to identify a brand or product.

Loyalty Program: A program that rewards customers who are members for their business and loyalty, designed to retain clients and keep them coming back to your spa or practice.

Machine Learning: A way to use data to improve computer performance for a set of tasks, not to be confused with AI.

Marketing Funnel: Illustrates the customer journey from awareness to purchase.

Memberships: Memberships are a promotional strategy, most common in spas and medspas, designed to offer more value to clients by curating offers on products and services that they are most interested in.

Meme: A symbol, image, video, or catchphrase turned into a graphic to be shared from person to person.

Meta: A new digital reality (short for Metaverse) that combines social media, AR, and VR to allow users to interact in an online digital world. Meta currently owns Facebook, Instagram, Messenger, and WhatsApp.

Meta Description: An HTML tag that provides a brief summary of a web page's content.

Metadata Tags: HTML tags that describe a web page's content and affect a website's ranking in search results.

Metrics: Marketing metrics are values used to measure marketing performance over time. A marketing metric might involve reach, engagement, lifetime value, or another indicator of success.

Mobile First: A model of website configuration used for narrow screen mobile devices like phones to work around the restrictions for mobile devices.

Modality: A high-level data category, such as numbers, text, images, video, or audio.

Multichannel Marketing: A marketing strategy used by brands and practices to define and communicate offers and marketing materials to customers across many channels, including websites, mobile, social media, direct mail, call centers, text messaging, email, outdoor advertising, etc.

Native Advertising: A type of promotional tactic that matches the style and format of an organic post. Ads are identifiable by a label that reads "sponsored" or "promoted" to distinguish native ads from more organic content.

Neural Network: A computer system designed to function like the human brain, also called a neural net.

Non-Fungible Token (NFT): A digital file like a JPEG of a piece of art, real estate, music, video, or other assets that are bought and sold online, sometimes with cryptocurrency. NFTs are unique, and no two NFTs are the same.

Omnichannel Marketing: A strategy that aligns content delivery across multiple marketing channels online and offline to provide a seamless, consistent experience for the target audience.

Open Assistant: A conversational AI chat-based technology that was intended for everyone to use.

Open Rate: A measurement to determine the percentage of subscribers who open a specific email out of your total number of subscribers.

Organic Content: Refers to free original content (not paid) that is shared on social media platforms including posts, videos, and stories which are used to elevate an individual or brand.

Outdoor Advertising: Marketing opportunities that reach the consumer while they are outside, including billboards, bus stops, kiosks, subways, airports, taxis, etc.

Outbound Marketing: The act of getting your messaging out into the marketplace to reach clients and potential customers. This can be accomplished in many ways including social media, advertising, email marketing, text messages, and any other tactic.

Paid Search: A type of digital marketing strategy that allows companies to pay search engines to place their ads higher on relevant search engine results pages (SERPs) with the goal of driving traffic to their site.

Pay Per Click (PPC): Adverts that target specific customers through sponsored links online.

Pinned Post: A pinned post is a social media post saved to the top of your page or profile on social media platforms to feature an important announcement or highlight your best content.

Podcast: A type of digital media, usually audio, that is available in a series of episodes or parts and is streamed or downloaded by users online.

Predictive Analytics: By combining data mining and machine learning, predictive analytics can forecast what will happen within a given timeframe based on historical data and trends.

Press Release: An official announcement, in the form of print or video, created to share with media outlets to spread news about a brand or company.

Prompt Engineering: Refers to the process of designing, refining, and optimizing input prompts to guide a generative AI model toward producing desired accurate outputs.

Prospect: A potential customer who has been qualified as meeting specific criteria which indicates an ability and likelihood to buy.

QR Code: A quick response code is a type of two-dimensional matrix barcode that is a machine-scannable image and can instantly be read using the camera on a smartphone.

Reputation Management: Influences on the reputation of a brand or individual. This can range from search results, reviews, ratings, media coverage, comments on social media channels, word of mouth, etc.

Responsive Design: Refers to how well your website can adjust to the screen size of visitors' devices, phones, websites, tablets, watches, etc. If the time is too long, the visitor may log out.

Retargeting: An online advertising strategy that is used to re-engage website visitors who have left a website without converting (i.e., making a purchase, filling out a form, posting a query). A small tracking tag is embedded in your website's code to target these prospects on other websites and social networks.

Return on Investment (ROI): Return on investment refers to the financial return of a marketing effort compared to the initial investment. ROI is calculated by subtracting the initial cost of investment from the proceeds of that investment and then dividing that sum by the initial cost of investment.

Search Engine Optimization (SEO): The strategic usage of keywords in website navigation, content, and inbound links to boost rankings for search results on platforms such as Google, Bing, etc.

SEM: Search engine marketing includes efforts to ensure that a business is displayed prominently on search engine results pages, such as Google and Bing. This includes both search engine optimization (SEO) and pay-per-click (PPC).

SERP: Search engine results page is the page that a search engine returns to after a user submits a search query. These usually include paid search and pay-per-click (PPC) ads.

Shadow Banning: Refers to blocking or partially blocking a user or the user's content online so that the user is not aware. Also referred to as stealth banning, hell banning, ghost banning, and comment ghosting.

Shopify: Global platform that is used by brands, practices, medspas, business owners, and creators to set up an online shop.

SMS: Short message service enables a mobile device to send, receive, and display messages of up to 160 characters. Messages received are stored in the network if the subscriber's device is inactive and are relayed when it becomes active.

Social Listening: The act of finding and assessing what is being said about a company, topic, brand, or person on social media channels. Taking action may include responding to a client's post and revising your social strategy.

Sponsored Post: Social media posts in which an influencer or celebrity highlights a brand or product that they have been paid to promote. These posts must be identified as ads using a hashtag like #ad or #sponsored.

Strong AI: Also referred to as General AI. The field of research focused on developing AI that is equal to the human mind in terms of ability.

Structured Data: Tabular data (for example, organized in tables, databases, or spreadsheets) that can be used to train some machine learning models. Unstructured data lacks a consistent format or structure (for example, text, images, and audio files) and requires more advanced techniques to extract insights.

Subscriptions: A promotional model that gives customers access to products and services or other perks for a set period.

Super App: An application that provides end users (customers, partners, or employees) with a set of core features plus access to independently created mini apps.

Survey: A collection of first-hand data from customers, vendors, stakeholders, or the general public. Market surveys are usually conducted to gather data so that better marketing, growth, and product decisions can be made.

Top of the Funnel (ToFu): Refers to tactics used to create awareness for a new product, treatment, location, etc. to generate brand awareness and leads in the market.

Upselling: The practice of guiding a customer to an upgraded version of a product, service, or something additional when he or she is about to buy.

User-Generated Content (UGC): Content that is created by a customer or patient in any form (reviews, testimonials, video, photos) that you can repurpose to elevate your brand.

Uniform Resource Locator (URL): A URL is an address used to identify an online resource, such as an HTML site or image.

User-Generated Content (UGC): Also abbreviated to UGC, user-generated content is the process of curating content from your followers and repurposing it for your own social media with credit.

Viral: Viral campaigns can lead to content being shared to huge audiences in a very short amount of time.

Virtual Reality (VR): Virtual reality is a simulated 3D environment that enables users to explore and interact with a virtual surrounding in a way that feels like it is reality.

Virtual Stores: An e-commerce experience powered by extended reality tools which aim to bridge the gap between digital and real-life shopping.

Voice Search: Using your voice for actionable tasks like search, directions, the weather, etc. via Siri, Alexa, Google Assistant, Cortana, and others.

Weak AI: Also referred to as Narrow AI, refers to AI that has a set range of skills and focuses on one particular set of tasks. Most AI in use is weak AI, meaning that they are unable to learn or perform tasks outside of their skill set.

White Paper: A backgrounder, list, or problem-solution format written to provide persuasive and factual evidence about a product, service, or method intended to influence the customer or buyer's decision.

Word-Of-Mouth Marketing (WOM): The oral or written advocacy of goods or services from a satisfied customer to a prospective customer.

Sources

https://www.telusinternational.com
https://www.wrike.com
https://www.hopperhq.com
https://www.wix.com
https://www.hubspot.com
https://www.hootsuite.com
https://www.mckinsey.com

Index

external agency, 54
fourteen government TikTok bans, 49–50
hashtag strategy, 62
important metrics and KPIs, 55
influencers, 64–65
Instagram Live, 53
Instagram Reels, 53
management platforms, 61
metrics to Tabs on, 55
newsflash, 63–64
popular channels by demographic, 58
posting best practices, 56
posting cadence, 57
posting patient photos, 58–59
reality check, 56
setting budget, 53–54
social selling to add revenue, 66
social strategy, 67
start with a plan, 57
strategies for social success, 57–58
tap into your community, 67
TikTok trends, 50–51
time is money, 51–52
tools you can use, 54
valuable platforms, 58
value of sharing real patient photos, 60
welcome TikTok creators, 50
where are they now, 48
working with influencers and creators, 64
Social selling, 66
Social trends for your marketing plan, 81
Solo practice, 1–2
Spammer, 21
Special perks, 12
Sponsored content, 60
Stanford University, 94
Start with a plan, 57
Stickers, 75, 76, 78
Stock images, 38–39
Storyteller, 37
Storytelling, 88
Strategies for social success, 4–5, 17, 57
Streamlining your business, 4
Subscription services, 12
Super apps, 80
Super helpful business tips for ten key channels, 81
Superintelligent AI, 95

T

Tabs, 55
Taking care of business, 36
Talking points, 76
Tap into your community, 67
Target audience, 38
Target the right audience, 15
Tech neck, 2
Techniques for retaining patients, 11
Technology, 30
Ten GIF tips, 89

Test and optimize, 16
Text, 84
Texting, 19–20
Text messaging, 19–20, 91, 92
    examples of CTAs, 91–92
    highest ROI platforms, 92
Think before posting, 57
Think global, act local, 22
Tiered pricing, 12
TikTok, 7, 14, 23, 49–51
TikTok-ing, 50
TikTok trends, 50–51
Time is money, 51–52
Tips for a beautiful channel, 72
Tips for working with creators, 36
Tools you can use, 43–44, 54
    AI help, 55
    external agency, 54
    social channels, 55
Touchpoints, 2, 7, 12
Tracking and evaluating, 21–22
Traditional marketing, 15
Traffic, 29
Traffic sources, 31
Treatment menu, 10
Trend alert, short-form videos, 86–87
Trending on Meta, 78
Trust factor, 15–16
Trustworthiness, 24
Twitter (X), 49, 108
Types of digital content
    images, 43
    text, 43
    video, 43

U

Ultimate endorsement, 60
Unique content strategy, 28
URL, 19, 72
User-generated content (UGC), 61
U.S. Federal Trade Commission, 21, 65
Using creators to elevate your brand, 36
Using video across all channels, 87–88

V

Valuable platforms, 58
Value of blogs, 40
Value of influencers, 34–35
Value of sharing real patient photos, 60
Value to treatments, 12–13
Ventura, 68
Video, 84
Virtual consults, xiii, 1–4
Virtual practice, 1
Virtual reality (VR), 78–79
Virtual stores, 80
Vision Pro, 68, 80
Voice search, 17, 94, 97